MW01282355

# Your Stress…

*and start nourishing your soul*

## Dina Hansen, NHD

ISBN:1495916456
ISBN-13:9781495916458

*To Mary,*
*may you live a*
*truly Nourishing life!*

"**The benefits I've received during this program allowed me to better manage my stress**, truly love and value myself and live a more fulfilling life filled with love, peace and happiness." -Christine M (Hand-in-Hand Coaching Client)

"**Without Dina's help, I would still be overwhelmed in a sea of doubt** waiting for my life to change with no plan or idea of HOW to change it. Now, I have a plan. I see improvement. I go after the things I want in my life. Dina has given me the lifelong skills and shown me how to use them to live the life I want." -Ann L. (Group Coaching & Hand-in-Hand Coaching Client)

"I would recommend you (Dina) to anyone that is looking to make more lifetime changes (rather than temporary changes) regarding food, weight and health. **Dina is fantastic at helping you get past the underlying causes and helping you to find your voice** and listen and trust your own body and intuition." -Stacey L. (Hand-in-Hand Coaching Client)

"**I think the most important thing is that Dina offers solutions. Practical solutions!** I'm a problem solver myself in my business life so I appreciate someone helping me. Now I have a more concentrated mind and true digestive relief" - Susie W. (Hand-in-Hand Coaching Client)

"**Working with Dr. Dina has taught me to really look at my food & enjoy it!** Instead of working on one facet of my life like my anxiety, we work on my whole person so that I can comfortably introduce new changes in my life that stick and last" -Linda L. (Group Coaching & Hand-in-Hand Coaching Client)

# DEDICATION

I would like to take this opportunity to thank all the women who have allowed me the privilege of working with them over the years. I believe there are no mistakes. You found me at a time when you were at a cross roads and knew the timing was right for you to metamorphasize from the old person you were, that was sick and tired of being sick & tired, to the person you've become, who is confident, mindful of her personal needs and aware of how to satisfy them. And I couldn't be prouder. I want to thank you for putting your mark on my life as well. You've helped me grow and evolve on just as many levels, and for that, I am eternally grateful.

I offer my gratitude, kisses and hugs to my husband for all his support & inspiration, to my daughter for always teaching me patience & joy, to my parents for never losing faith in me and I want to thank YOU for trusting your instincts and choosing to awaken and develop a whole new relationship with your food, yourself and your life.

Always seek within to find the solution that is the right fit for you.

Namaste`
Dina

# CONTENTS

Introduction

## AUTHOR'S NOTE:

This book is in no way a replacement for any medical advice. To the contrary, it is to be used as a companion to your current healthcare choices, and any current therapies.

Information contained within this book is for educational purposes only and you are encouraged to take full responsibility for your choices and actions as they will empower your ability to heal in mind, body & soul.

So please be true to you.

*"When we are true to ourselves, all that is toxic and burdensome, simply falls away"*
-Dina Hansen, NHD

# DON'T READ THIS INTRODUCTION...
## *IT'S PERSONAL*

Now that I have your attention, I would like to thank you for choosing this book. A book is a very personal thing, and I'm honored that you wanted to include this particular book (and me) into your library and your life.

At some point in our lives, we've all experienced stress and anxiety along with all of its various debilitating effects to our health physically, mentally or emotionally. My personal experience with stress & anxiety was pretty extreme, and the eye-opening journey took me from feeling over-whelmed, out of control and out of my mind, to a place of inner peace, mindful awareness and total control. My transformation is what inspired me to help women achieve a greater level of awareness, self-care, inner peace and balance. One of the things I've come to realize, through years of observation and education, is that we all experience stress in our own very unique way. Maybe you'll be able to relate to the story I'm about to share with you, maybe you've experienced some of the same feelings, thoughts or physical pains. Then again, maybe you're reading this simply because you are curious and the title intrigued you, but you're really very healthy and nothing really makes you stressed at all. Let's find out.....

IT'S MY STORY...and I'm sticking to it!

I grew up in a middle-class home on Long Island. Both of my parents tended to be perfectionists, had high expectations and repressed a lot of worry, anxiety, stress & tension. I was loved and cared for, but being the sensitive person that I am, all that stress & tension rubbed off on me pretty easily, and affected me more deeply than anyone knew.

My father worked by day as a music teacher, went to school part-time at night during the week to become a school administrator, and played gigs at night on weekends in NYC to support us. My mother was a full-time speech pathologist in an elementary school who did her best to excel at her job, and always did her best to be there for my sister and me whenever we needed her. Just like many households today… maybe even yours.

Yet because of their busy schedules, when I was about 10, my sister and I were on our own for a couple of hours after school. This meant we had the run of the house and could eat & do anything we wanted. Talk about FREEDOM! Left to our own devices, we lazed around the house ingesting as many sweets and artificial foods that we could. We ate chocolate milk powder right out of the container, sometimes with peanut butter, sometimes without. We consumed cookies, candy, pastries, canned pasta and a variety of other processed foods until our mother came home from work. What kid wouldn't? After all, we were tired and wanted to kick-back after a full day of school. We needed to rest & recharge. We wanted to feel good. So, we did what anyone might do in that situation; we gorged ourselves on sweets and comfort food until we felt happy and relaxed again.

After a few weeks of this free-for-all, I began having uncontrollable cravings for sweets every moment of every day. In fact, it was on my mind so frequently, that it was almost all I could think about. I was constantly planning out or plotting when and how I was going to get my next sweet treat. Before I knew it, those sweets became my haven. My personal solace for when I thought I had no one to turn to when I felt anxious, stressed-out or depressed. I believed that sweets were the one thing in my life that would make everything all right, even if it was only for a little while. My sugar habit went on for years, with my dependency on it constantly growing. In fact, at one point, it got so critical, I would stuff sugar packets into my pants pockets or my bra so I could have "a fix" when I needed to feel good or have a shot of "energy". It eventually came with me to college, as the trusted best friend I made it out to be. However, it turned out to be my worst enemy.

I went to college to receive a bachelors in elementary education. One, because my parents lead me that direction, and Two, because I love little kids and we often get along with each other very easily. However, when I got there, I discovered that going away to college was much more than just a place to escape my parents and have a good time. Suddenly, I began to realize that I had new responsibilities and had to deal with the pressures of juggling my very full class schedule, homework, practicals, and my ever important social life. Sometimes I would get so busy, I would forget to eat or put off eating, so I could get my work done, then feel ravenous and moody later in the day. So to help me cope, my trusty comfort food was with me every step of the way. Self medicating with sweets was the most inexpensive, quick fix I found to give me the illusion of control. Very often I would go to the vending machine to grab a couple of candy bars and a Coke as a convenient "on-the-go meal" for my breakfast or lunch if there was no time to head to the cafeteria. I drank coffee light & sweet, mostly because it tasted like ice cream that way, and I drank it as often as I could, because it gave me the surge of energy I needed during the day to get stuff done. If I wanted to relax in the evening, I'd have several beers, shots, or wine coolers with my friends at parties or even just play drinking games while watching TV.

And yes, I know what you're thinking; "This sounds like a typical college experience. Everyone does this." Maybe they do. However, for me, the slow drip of my own constant worry, anxiety, low self-esteem and internal conflicts, combined with the years of malnourishment from all the sweets and processed foods I'd consumed, was just too much. My body & mind couldn't take any more.

The sad part is, that they had been sending me subtle signals for years that I was hurting myself. Only I had been stubbornly and naively ignoring them; tuning them out and pushing throughout the pain, instead of listening to it and finding a solution beyond the surface.

Some of these signals seemed to be nothing. For example, I often felt fuzzy brained & light headed, or totally hyper with my mind racing all over the place, which made it hard to concentrate. I'd feel such extreme changes in moods from happy-go-lucky to manic depressive within moments of each other, that I would think self-berating, hateful thoughts about myself and compare myself to others mercilessly. I'd sometimes see "stars" as I was walking to class, and would usually just blow it off, thinking the sun was probably in my eyes or chalk it up to being over-tired. The constant dull ache in my knees I developed, carried over from childhood, would sometimes make it incredibly painful to walk, especially going up and down the mountainous hillside of the beautiful Vermont campus I was attending.

Gradually it began to get worse. After eating, my stomach started to have more regular pains, often with the sharp sting of reflux or a constant bloating feeling. I would often cry in my room, all by myself in deep despair & constant worry over things I couldn't put my finger on and wish I was dead. I did my best to hide my internal pain & suffering from those around me for a very long time. I'd put on a happy-faced mask and pretended that all was good with the world. And why wouldn't I? Especially at that age? After all, who'd want to hang out with someone who was depressed, anxious and only thinks the worst about themselves all the time? And I even believed I had to pretend that life was fabulous, even around my family. And believe me; I got <u>very good</u> at camouflaging what was going on inside the private, intimate hell I was living within. Then one day, during a ballet class, my mask began to crack, and hiding my secret became more difficult.

We were practicing pirouettes across the floor, and suddenly, I just dropped to the ground. I lost consciousness and fainted. When I regained consciousness, I was mortified. Nevertheless, I laughed it off saying that I just got dizzy because I wasn't focusing like I was supposed to be. I ignored it, pushed it aside from my mind, stuffed down my fear and continued on with the class as if it was nothing. However, it was something.

My body & mind had continued to send me louder and louder messages that my lifestyle and eating habits were not nourishing me as the weeks went on. Signals that I needed to start making changes, and now. Yet, I had refused to listen and the lesson of a lifetime was gaining momentum and steamrolling straight towards me.

The final straw was the night I came back from class, and unlocked my dorm room door, as usual. I put the key in the keyhole, and then before I knew what was happening, my body felt like jelly, and everything went dark. From what I was told, I had suddenly dropped to the ground, and went into a full blown, grand-mal seizure right in there in the doorway. And everyone on the dorm floor watched, UGH! I lost consciousness just as I did in ballet class, except this time my whole body convulsed aggressively, and my eyes rolled back into my head. There was no escaping it now. There was no blowing it, pushing it aside or laughing it off. The ambulance was on its way and I needed serious help.

Soon after that episode, and several more like it, I was dismissed from school for medical reasons. I was sent back home for several rounds of neurological testing at NYU medical, only for the doctors and specialists to have no conclusive answers as to what caused my episodes. They were only able to conclude that I wasn't epileptic. One specialist even suggested that my episodes were psychosomatic, which made me furious at the time. I mean, why and how would I "think" myself into having something like that happen to me? Especially something, that was so public & embarrassing! After getting incredibly frustrated with this prognosis and tired of the various effects I was having from the multitude of medications prescribed to me over the months, I decided to take charge of my life and do something about it myself.

Even though I didn't like what that one doctor said about my thoughts creating my convulsions, a small nagging part of me thought maybe he was onto something. It was so uncomfortable to think about, that I decided to look into it further, because nothing else was making sense or helping to make be better.

See, back in High School, I had a teacher who once told me that, "We all create our own reality". I figured that maybe, on some level, I actually did create this. I wondered what would happen if I observed my thoughts, my habits and my lifestyle. And could I change something that wasn't helping me be the healthy person I thought I was by doing this? I mean, what I had been doing wasn't working for me, so what did I have to lose? Right?!

Gradually, with the help of careful self-experimentation, research and ongoing education, I transformed my old ways of thinking about myself, the ways I perceived stress as well as my coping mechanisms. I uncovered answers that were definitely "outside the box" of typical western thinking. After receiving my Doctorate in Natural

Health, with a specialization in mind/body medicine, I was in a fortunate position to be trained by some of most well respected physicians and leading wellness experts in the world when it comes to integrative and mind/body medicine. Doctors such as Dr. Walter Willett (who is the Chair of Harvard University's Department of Nutrition), Dr. Deepak Chopra (world-renowned mind/body healing pioneer) and Dr. Neal Barnard (founding president of the Physicians Committee for Responsible Medicine), to name a few. I studied energy medicine, the healing power of wholistic nutrition and the beautiful mind/body connection that unconsciously drives our actions. The best part though, was the understanding that I could take what I had learned over the years, and help other women suffering with anxiety, low self-esteem and emotional eating issues transform their lives-only a lot more simply and a lot more quickly than I did. Because now I had the knowledge of how to cut a path through the clutter, all the over-whelming information and go straight to the heart of what creates a true metamorphosis.

Once upon a time, bread, sweets and processed foods were my crutch, my solace, and the rug to cover up emotions I didn't want to deal with. Now, they're only a sometime food, because my deep craving for them dissolved very naturally. I'm a lot pickier about what goes into my body & my mind now. I learned that I'm worth taking the time & energy to be selective. It's worth my peace of mind to make decisions that feel good to me, instead of what I think others expect of me. I've learned to tune into my unique needs and mindfully fulfill them…and so have my clients.

## WHY YOU NEED TO READ THIS BOOK

I must admit, when I set out to write this book it was initially written with the intention of being a way to put everything I've learned together in one place, as a way to share this information with my clients. A tool available only to my personal clients, and a resource for others interested in working with me. However, a gentle nudge from a good friend of mine encouraged me to write this book so women all over the world could start making significant shifts in their lives, at their pace, with a bit of guidance from someone who's been there. A series of personal coaching sessions of sorts, in your purse.

It's my intention to permanently change your relationship with yourself, your food and your stress. Therefore, each step of the way, I'll be providing opportunities for you to experiment with what I'm teaching in your own life. So instead of just reading the book, getting some information and going back to your old ways of doing things (that obviously don't seem to be working), I'll be coaching you with real life, practical suggestions. So Take your time through each coaching session. Think of this book as your portable coach; an effective tool to help you unload the mindless, self-sabotaging habits that have become such a monkey on your back over the years.

Within each coaching session, I'll share the same mindful stress solutions I teach the women I work with in person. Steps that have proven effective in creating a higher quality of life and are self-nurturing, balancing & lasting.

You don't have to decide this now, but I highly suggest teaming up with a friend, or forming your own supportive inner circle. Knowing we are supported and are being held accountable for our actions, especially in the beginning, can mean the difference between just "trying something new" and choosing a new lifestyle. Just knowing that someone we trust is counting on us to make choices that are good for us can help us become more to consistent in practicing what we're learned. According to my clients, accountability is one of the greatest tools they receive when working with me, whether they are private hand-in-hand clients or clients' part of a Group Coaching Program. So if you have a friend, or several friends, that you can count on to be supportive, honest and reliable to keep each other on task without judgement, please buddy-up! Remember, when it comes to life, one size does not fit all. Each one of us is unique and has our own set of unique needs physically, mentally and emotionally. What may be healthy for one person may not be healthy to another. So tune in and discover what nourishes you. Follow the advice of your inner guide, and play with those suggestions.

So many people take a very serious approach to reducing stress and anxiety, not to mention healthy eating. I am here to be different from the rest and encourage you to PLAY WITH YOUR FOOD!

So, before I end this introduction, I'd like to thank you for making the choice to be good to yourself. For taking the opportunity to plant the seeds to another way of living that could be much more nourishing and satisfying than the life you're living now.

I believe that if we can be taught to think poorly about ourselves, to live with anxiety and fear, then we can learn to crowd out those old learnings with new teachings that are much more uplifting, empowering and freeing.

What if all it took was one empowering step at a time to create the nourishing life of our dreams? What if instead of forcing ourselves to do things we think we "should", we simply did them because they felt right and were a priority for us? What if we could look back over a year or so and be able to witness the transformation in our thoughts our actions had on our lives ... and smile with a deep sense of satisfaction?

# Coaching Session 1:
## *The Mind/Body Connection*
## *& Cravings*

Ok, so I'm about to state the obvious here; we all eat. Yet, what triggers us to eat, especially with the stressed out, busy lifestyle so many of us are living these days? Is it because we honestly have a feeling of hunger, or are we experiencing boredom from the mundane routine of our lives? Do we need some comfort during all this stress, or do we just want to feel more in control, when everything seems to be careening away from us in utter chaos? Whatever our reasons, no matter who we are, we all experience stress, and eventually we all eat. Many times finding ourselves mindlessly over eating, completely unaware of the actual food or food-like substances we are putting into our mouths. All too often, stress and cravings are the instigators.

At times, we'll even go without eating, simply to get things done. Then find ourselves famished later on during the day, and can't figure out why we don't have the energy to keep up with our kids, why we aren't losing that muffin top, or why we need all those cups of coffee and sweet snacks during the day. This is yet another affect of stress. When we are stressed, we tend to neglect our needs and ourselves. Which creates cravings later on in the day for things we wouldn't ordinarily choose to eat, especially in the quantity we seem to eat them, if we weren't feeling so insane at the moment from stress, and a lack of nourishment. According to one of the medical dictionaries I've been going through recently, a food craving is defined as "An intense, urgent, or abnormal desire or longing to consume something". Sounds pretty accurate to me...

You and I know, when we feel stressed-out and emotionally overwhelmed, it can trigger an intense craving for something to take away that suffering. When it does, it seems that NOTHING is going to satisfy us like what we yearning for! It doesn't matter if were craving salty chips, sweet chocolate, alcohol or a combination of all three at once. When we want it, it's like a drug, and we'll stop at nothing until we get it! Many of the foods we crave when we're in a highly emotional state, are actually highly addictive. Foods like those that contain sugar, caffeine, monosodium glutamate (MSG), vinegar, and certain spices which make us crave more of them even after we just finished eating a whole bag. And we have those cravings for a reason. Our body/mind is telling us that we are lacking something to help us stay balanced. A sugar craving could mean that your body is needing more energy or glucose for better brain function, or a lack of minerals such as chromium, zinc or magnesium. A salty craving could be a way of your body telling you that you're needing more water because you're dehydrated. It is also an indication that your adrenal glands (stress glands) are overworked and maxed out, you need to take a breather. We lose vital minerals during stress and a salt craving is one way that your body attempts to replenish them. Fried, fatty food cravings are your body's way of telling you that you are lacking chromium. Although your body only needs small trace amounts of it, it's one of the most important minerals in the body. After all, it's vital to the metabolism of glucose, for maintaining blood sugar and helps greatly with people prone to depression. Dr. Andrew Saul, is a great resource if you want to learn more about how vitamins can replace many over the counter drugs.

Our "intense urgent desire" shows us the powerful mind/body connection. And they are intricately connected. Our thoughts can cause a reaction within our body and our biological state can have an effect on our mental state. Just think about the last thing that really made you laugh out loud.  Remember where you were, who you were with and how it felt to be with them in that moment. I bet it just put a smile on your face, didn't it? Maybe even a little chuckle escaped your lips. Did you notice that you may have breathed a bit deeper as you were remembering those good times? Along the same lines of thinking, our thoughts can also powerfully create cravings just by thinking about something we have an emotional connection to. In fact, some nutritional researchers in the North East have recently been researching physical cravings and their connection to the mind. What they discovered was that food cravings can be an expression of addiction, and many of the processed foods we crave, affect both body and mind in some very interesting ways.

*Check it out...*

If we're one of the millions of Americans who follow the Standard American Diet (otherwise known as SAD), we tend to eat large quantities of pre-packaged, convenient, fast foods. Especially when we're feeling stressed-out, overwhelmed or depressed. These foods rob our bodies of the nutrients we need for optimal biological functioning, interferes with how our body uses essential nutrients, and actually creates internal stress & cravings. Does that surprise you? The science that constructs these foods, simply cannot reproduce the same level of balanced nourishment Mother Nature has expertly created for thousands of years. All those food-like substances created in laboratories set the stage for bad moods, fatigue, weight gain and increased stress levels due to their lack of nutrient balance.

Here's something else that's fairly interesting, these same researchers discovered that sugar addiction can be connected to a person needing more sweetness in one's life. Or, as the Italians say, "la dolce vita" the sweet life. With the fast paced, rush, rush, get it done, and show it off lifestyle many of us are living, I would agree, wouldn't you? Imagine what we would avoid eating and over-eating, if we simply learned how to enjoy life's little pleasures. If we simply slowed down enough to even taste our food from the first bite, to the last.

Say you're not a sweets kind of person? You like diving into a bag of those chips and salty snacks instead? Well, those same researchers discovered that people who tend to eat foods loaded with MSG, such as chips, dips, and other such processed foods, could mean you're looking for more excitement in life. Many times these same people are eating out of sheer boredom and don't know what to do to entertain themselves. Could that be you?

**Kind of puts a new perspective on cravings doesn't it?**

The kicker is, if we ignore signals from our body telling us we need real nourishment (on our plates & in our lives), we're more likely to over-think, over-react, and over-eat than we will when we're truly satiated. When we receive the nutrients we need physically, mentally & emotionally, we become more balanced naturally, without ever having to force ourselves into submission with will-power.

Cravings come in both the biological form, and the emotional form. Many times the foods we crave and eat for comfort, are the very foods our mother, or caregiver, offered us as children to soothe us when we were hurt or upset. Therefore, it makes sense that those are the foods we would gravitate to as adults when feeling overwhelmed, stressed, depressed or struggling with any other uncomfortable emotion. Yet through it all, our body/mind always seeks homeostasis. This incredibly intelligent body we walk around with, always knows what we need to thrive. Unfortunately though, we're the ones who tend to sabotage this natural phenomenon, by either letting our emotions overwhelm us and sucking us down into the abyss, or consciously instructing ourselves to do something else (such as, eat later).

Because our body/mind is so accommodating, it follows our instructions, and does its best to adapt to what we throw at it, until it can take no more. That's when aches, pains and crazy cravings really are hard to ignore. It's our body's way of yelling at us that what we are doing isn't working! We need a better source of nourishment in order to function more harmoniously. Choosing to starve our body/mind of the very things it needs to thrive, let alone, to be able to better handle our stress, doesn't work. In the long run, it only makes things worse.

Think of the last time you skipped breakfast. Maybe you didn't eat until noon or much later. Didn't things start to get a little out of your control the longer you went without eating? Maybe you experienced fatigue and had a hard time focusing on your tasks. Maybe your temper got short and you started thinking irrational thoughts. Being more aware of the signals our body/mind gives us that we're needing nourishment physically, mentally or emotionally really helps us prevent crazy cravings, and is fabulous at preventing stress and anxiety from getting out of control.

When we begin by paying attention to the tastes we crave, we start having a better understanding of what we are needing for true nourishment, instead of mindlessly reaching for habitual foods.

**When was the last time you payed attention to the tastes you crave?**

25

All food can be divided into 5 Tastes: Sweet, Salty, Sour, Spicy & Bitter

Which one do you crave more often?
Which one do you eat least?
What emotion are you feeling while you crave that taste?

## Take a Mindful Moment:

Before I go any further, I'm going to ask you to take the next 24-48 hours to find the answers to the questions above. Many times the foods we eat most often are symbolic of what we are craving in our lives, both nutritiously and emotionally. Helping us better understand where we are overloaded, and where we are malnourished. For example, I had a client who tended to ignore her cravings for greens because she had such a bad association with them. Every time she imagined eating some type of green, she felt queasy and immediately recalled her mother's limp broccoli sitting on the table, then told she wasn't allowed to leave until her father saw her consume everything on her plate. As a result, as an adult, instead of eating the greens she knew were good for her, she would eat lots of chocolate. When I suggested that her cravings for greens (a bitter taste) could be satisfied with DARK organic chocolate, at least 70%, she became excited and started to eat the dark chocolate instead.

Now I agree with you, greens would have been a better choice. However looking ahead at long term, positive change, we need to understand that it's all about gradual transition in the beginning stages of the game. DARK chocolate is one of the most delicious sources of antioxidants that we can enjoy guilt free. It's actually quite nutritious, rich with soluble fiber, iron, magnesium, copper, manganese, potassium, selenium, and phosphorous. Pretty cool, right? With her negative connection to greens, a higher quality substitute for her addiction was the best option. When we choose foods that are higher in quality, our satisfaction last longer, without robbing us of what we need to thrive in the first place. Plus, we get that positive emotional feedback we're craving as well!

*Now it's your turn...*

For the next 24-48 hours, simply be aware of your personal emotion-food connection. When you are feeling frustrated or angry what taste do you crave? How is that different from when you feel sad or lost? And what happens when you satisfy your craving with higher quality foods, versus pre-processed, low quality foods?

**Step1**-Check in with yourself-Be aware of your current experience & your state of mind. Be fully present in your experience and see if you can label what emotion you are feeling without attaching any meaning or reason behind it.

**Step 2**-Now that you've identified what emotion you're feeling, what taste are you yearning for? Sweet, Salty, Sour, Pungent or Bitter? So for example many times when we are tired or stressed we yearn for something bitter like chocolate or coffee.

**Step 3-**Imagine tasting that food on your tongue. As it is chewed and swallowed, imagine how you feel afterwards? Are you feeling satiated and nourished or temporarily subdued and a bit lacking or empty inside? Trust what comes up first, without second guessing yourself. Your instincts are more accurate than you may be giving them credit for.

**Step 4**-Ask yourself what higher quality, natural food would satiate you and maintain satisfaction longer? The list of *Natural Food Options* below each taste will help you figure that out. After you eat, be aware of how you feel 10,15-30 minutes after you eat. How do you feel in body & mind?

*I suggest keeping a small journal* with you either on your phone or on a small notebook in your purse. Studies show that when we write down what we eat, and record the effects they have on us, we have a better understanding of how our foods affect us. My clients typically receive a handout with this available to them in their Transformation Toolbox. However you can easily do this yourself by keeping track of the feeling you felt, the taste you craved, the food you chose and the result afterwards.

Below is an abbreviated list of Natural Food Options to help you exchange some higher quality choices for the processed ones you may have eaten in the past.

**Sweet**-When we worry a lot, and need more sweetness, love, joy and compassion in life, we gravitate towards sweet foods. Instead, think about what makes you feel playful & happy. Whom can you call for support? Where can you get a good hug?

Natural Food Options: fruit, root vegetables, squash, corn on the cob, local honey, real maple syrup

**Salty**-Why let fear get the best of you (FEAR= False Evidence Appearing Real)? What would you like to happen instead?

Natural Food Options: buckwheat, kidney or pinto beans,kale, water chestnuts, wakame (seaweed), pickles, sesame seeds, chia seeds, blackberries, cranberries, watermelon, scallops, crab, lobster, squid and pork

**Sour**-When we are feeling impatient, feel angry and tend to shout at everyone, we tend to want sour foods. Instead of being a sour puss, and stressing out those around you as well as yourself, practice deep breathing and a little patience.

Natural Food Options: oats, barley, peanuts, split peas, broccoli, zucchini, green peas, Boston lettuce, romaine or Bibb lettuce, cashews, avocado, grapefruit, lemons or limes, sour cream, yogurt, trout, chicken, sauerkraut and seitan

**Bitter**-When we feel a bit stuck, and having trouble circulating through life, we tend to go for bitter foods like coffee (which can overload the adrenals after a while if we consume too much). Imagine instead what it would be like on the other side of what's holding you back. How great could it be? What would you see, hear and feel if you could have the outcome you desired?

Natural Food Options: popcorn, amaranth, dandelion root or greens, escarole, okra, tomato, apricot, strawberry, raspberry, sesame seeds, sunflower seeds, pistachios, dark chocolate and shrimp.

Pungent, Spicy, Hot-These tastes are often associated with grief or sadness. Sometimes we go through a phase of personal growth and have a hard time letting go of who we once were, so we unconsciously gravitate to spicy foods. Sometimes it's sadness or grief for other reasons. Imagine how life would be if you just let go and moved forward with peace in your heart. How could you honor yourself (and anyone else this is associated with)?

Natural Food Options: rice, red chili pepper, daikon, celery, garlic, ginger, watercress, turnip greens, basil, clove, cinnamon, nutmeg, fennel, dill, horseradish, walnuts, hickory nut, egg whites, cod, flounder, halibut, turkey, mint, peppermint, spirulina, and tempeh.

## COACHING SESSION 2:
### *Goodbye Willpower*

WELCOME BACK...

Did you actually do the steps in the last section, or are you just reading on, telling yourself you'll try to do it later? You know the moment we say the word "try" we pre-suppose failure, and we sabotage any possible success we may have. We're actually telling the part of mind that determines our behavior, that we instead of doing what we said we would "try" to do, we aren't actually going to do it. Naturally as your coach, I want you to succeed. So go ahead, do the steps above.

I'll be here when you get back….

Did you really do it this time?

Fabulous!

So what did you learn from your Mindful Moment? What tastes did you discover you crave more often and how did they match-up with your state of mind? Then, what happened when you replaced your "usual" with a Natural Food Option?

If you struggled with this type of awareness, understand that this is great first step. Simply being *aware* that you are having trouble, actually tells us that you are consciously learning to make new habits. Keep it up. Just like everything else, with consistency and conscious practice, it will become second nature to you before you know it. Just like tying your shoe or walking. I believe in you and know you can do it, the question is, do you believe in yourself as well?

Sometimes, when we have cravings, we attempt to ignore them all together, thinking we'll depend on our "willpower" to muscle through them with the intention of getting more done or to lose weight. However, in my experience, this often backfires and only creates crazy, mindless, bingeing later on. Has that ever happened to you too?

The intention is in the right place, but the result is the exact opposite of what we wanted in the first place! Because skipping meals stresses your body out. It goes into starvation mode and begins to store fat. And we get bummed out, feeling like we just "failed" at something all over again! So a new wave of self-disappointment takes over, maybe even triggering us to eat more.

So many of us talk about "not having enough willpower" to explain away our reasons for eating that piece of cake, the donuts or even the chips. We blame "not having enough willpower" on why we didn't stick with our new workout routine, our new diet or anything else that seemed to fall off course according to our grand plans...

So, what would really happen if we suddenly "lost our willpower"?

Would we go running through the streets doing whatever we wanted? Looting bakery's, steeling car's, kissing random people?

Probably not...

Yet many of us do believe that without "willpower" we would end up lounging around all day, becoming couch potatoes, doing nothing except eating bon-bon's, watching TV, sleeping or whatever else tickles our lazy bones. However, when we use the excuse that we "lost our willpower" what we're essentially saying is that whatever it was that we needed our willpower for in the first place, really wasn't a priority for us, because we needed to force ourselves to do it.

Think about it for a moment. Would you ever have to force yourself to cuddle with your child when they were crying and needed you; or force yourself to accept a generous raise that was being handed to you? Probably not. Your child's well-being is a priority to you. Having more money to be able to better support yourself and your family is a priority. It's the reason we would take action without question.

What's a priority for you? What would you do without thinking, questioning or forcing yourself to do it, simply because it was THAT important to you?

Is it taking care of those you love? What about finding a way of soothing your emotions, especially when upset? And when was the last time you made self-care and compassion your priority?

Look, we can't escape eating. Food is essential to our survival and at the center of almost all life events. Sometimes we make healthy choices, sometimes we make less than stellar choices. That's just part of how life ebbs and flows. Having a bit of self-compassion instead of self-judgement is a big help here. Because when self-care is our priority, the need for us to rely so heavily on our will-power becomes less of an issue.

The moment you're aware that you made a "poor choice" notice if the decision came from your gut or your head. Very often our so-called, "lack of willpower" is coming from the memory voice of what someone said to us once before, or what we habitually tell ourselves through our own self-judgement, stemming from personal beliefs of inadequacy. This can also be true of what we hear in our heads AFTER we made a "poor choice". It might come in the form of scolding ourselves, berating ourselves or even packed with "should have" comments. Which honestly only sabotages our efforts to take more positive actions to help ourselves in the future. And yet, when we make a choice based on what is a priority or most important to us, there's no need for inner conversations. The choice comes from the heart or from your gut. It feels right and taking action simply becomes "a no-brainer".

Here's an example of what I'm talking about. A friend of mine told me a story about her sister, who was a teacher. She was very confident in her skills professionally, but extremely shy socially around her peers. She dreaded going out socially because she always felt inadequate in conversations that didn't involve anything to do with work. She was very passionate about what she did for a living, and enjoyed spending time with some of the people she worked with during the short lunch breaks she got. She wanted to go out socially with some of them but din't feel confident in saying anything. She was scared of being rejected and yet it was important to her because she really felt like she connected with them at school. She didn't socialize very much because she was so shy and had only lived in that state for a year, so she didn't have many friends. One day she was enjoying a good laugh with one of the women at work and the moment just felt right. So she very bravely asked if the other woman wanted to get together after work. And to her relief the other woman agreed. Since that first brave step, the two friends have become almost inseparable.

Over the years, I've discovered that what's most important to us, can often be linked to *why* we eat as well.

So, let's talk a little bit about <u>why</u> we eat. Because it isn't always for the reason we think.

At some point in our lives, we may have read or heard that food is fuel for the body. Food is not emotion. It's just a source of nourishment to give us the energy we need to function optimally.

My clients and I would disagree.

Both myself and the women I've worked over with the years chose to self medicate with food, because of the comfort and control food provided us in that moment. What's important to be aware of though, is that food alone is not emotion. <u>We</u> attach emotional connections to our food, and from those attachments, we create many of our addictions, then call them "comfort food". Which is one of the reasons why we seem to rely so heavily on the excuse of "not having any will-power" when we fall off the wagon of yet another diet. Our priority when we're down-in-the-dumps or feel overwhelmed is to receive comfort from a reliable source and have control over something. It has less to do with will-power. In fact most people who do diet frequently have more self control than their counterparts, they just aren't giving themselves the credit for it, because their inner critic won't let them.

To add to our dependance on "comfort-food" the foods we usually choose when out of sorts, is often processed food-like-substances made by companies we've grown-up with. Brands we identify with the comforts of home. These man-made products contain ingredients that create biochemical, and neurological addictions no different from the numerous toxic affects drugs, alcohol or tobacco have on us. What's worse is that many well known and trusted companies intentionally put these ingredients in their products to create an addiction. These trusted companies will then spend millions of dollars conducting research to learn how to better activate our triggers through these ingredients and advertising to make more money from our purchases. So no matter what their ads may tell us about how much they care, through their images, words and slick marketing, their interest is really focused on the bottom line: Not yours.

Let's break this down....
Companies make fake foods with addictive, toxic ingredients designed to make us crave their products. They spend millions of dollars on powerful, repetitive marketing and branding getting us to trust them. We come along with our stressed-out lifestyle, and our emotional needs, and BAM! We're hook like junkies!

No wonder we have a hard time breaking free from our addiction to these foods!

Have no fear though, there is a better way. A more natural way to satisfy those cravings for sweet, salty, fatty, sour, spicy, and bitter foods. Mother Nature is here and she genuinely has our best interests at heart. She knows that food is meant to be delicious, colorful and completely nourishing to our bodies and minds. She gives us the exact balance of satisfaction, nutrients and tastes that we need, in its own beautiful packaging, and hard to become addicted to when eaten in their natural state. Ahhhhhh... stress free simplicity!

Have you ever thought about this...our emotional connection to food, was actually developed at birth.

Think about it for a moment.

It all started right from the beginning with the comfort, safety and love of our mother as she nursed us as new born's and infants. As we got older, that emotional connection was cultivated through the feeding games our mother or father played with us as toddlers. As we grew, our mom might have offered us a cookie, an ice cream or sweet snack if we got hurt to help take away the pain. Then try as we might as adults, we just can't seem to shake that emotional connection to certain foods, and start telling ourselves we just can't stay away from them because we have no willpower.

What would happen, do you think, if the comfort food that was given to us as children was a carrot instead of a cookie? Where she would have played a game with the carrot to make us laugh instead of cry when we were hurt. It's still a deeply sweet taste, just natural and nutritionally balanced. Would that have made us crave carrots, like we crave cookies, or would we simply be able to appreciate & enjoy their sweet nourishment on a multitude of levels, instead of hating our vegetables?

Think for a moment about the foods you crave for comfort. You know, the one's that you think you need all your "will-power" to fight against having when you're on yet another restrictive diet.

What happens if I mention the smell of fresh-baked cookies fresh from the oven? What image came to your mind? What feelings popped up? What if I mention chocolate? Mac n' cheese? Peanut Butter and Jelly? What's the memory you have attached to those foods?

We crate attachments to these foods and their comforting memories. Then when we feel stressed out, or overwhelmed, we seek that feeling of safety from the past to soothe us. And the easiest way to find it again is to have the food that most easily triggers those feelings for us. Ever find yourself nervous about attending a social event, then she you get there, find you're gravitating towards certain foods like breads, cheeses, or pasta dishes? As an introverted person, I found I did that a lot more than I thought I did when I started paying attention to my actions and asking myself what thoughts I was thinking to make me feel take this action.

As I mentioned earlier, food is the center of all life's events; every celebration, social activity, business function and debate. It's even all over the media from books, magazines and newspapers to movies, the web and T.V.! Moreover, we tend to feel so passionate about our food, that the emotional connection we have with it, eventually becomes intricately connected with how we feel about ourselves. If we eat what we "should be eating" in the portion sizes we "must be choosing" we allow ourselves to feel good about ourselves and our choices. If we deny ourselves the tastes we crave, because it's not on the pre-planned menu for this week's diet, we find ourselves binging on everything else later on! Maybe even berating ourselves and ending up feeling worthless. Which triggers the belief that we are less than perfect, so we embark on another diet, and the cycle continues.

Over the years, I've learned that we tend to knead our emotions into everything we eat, just like we would knead bread dough before we set it to rise. As we do, we're absorbing those feeling deeper into our cells, feelings of shame, guilt and regret, or satisfaction, love and joy, and it changes our constitution. In 1994, Dr. Marasu Emoto from Japan, conducted a study where he would talk to water in either a mean and hateful way, or a tender, loving or compassionate way, then froze the water and studied it under a microscope. What he discovered was astounding. When he spoke with harsh words, the water crystals were disfigured and formed "angry" shapes. In fact, when you look through his book, *The Hidden Messages in Water,* you'll see that one of samples even looked like two soldiers pointing guns at each other! However, when he spoke with kindness and compassion to the water, the crystals formed into some of the most magical and beautiful shapes you could imagine. This is a perfect demonstration of how our thoughts and words affect us. Think about this for a moment, we are about 85% water-how are your thoughts affecting you? What emotions are you solidifying into your cells every time you eat and what would happen if you focused on self appreciation, love and gratitude instead of self judgment, persecution and guilt?

The next time you sit down to a meal take a moment and ask yourself, "What emotions am I feeding myself right now?". In the ancient Japanese healing art Jin Shin Jyutsu, we learn that emotions become attitudes when we become attached to them, and forget to let them go. Many of us feed on the attitudes Worry, Fear, Anger, Grief or Pretense all day long without ever realizing it, creating more suffering for ourselves.

If we're focused on any of these attitudes while eating, we make them more powerful, and disrupt healthy digestion. On the other hand, if we are focused on our blessings as we eat, we may find ourselves more relaxed and happier with less digestive complaints and stress afterwards. And again, this eliminates the need for willpower. There is no more fight, only peace within and love.

We all know that when we feel good about ourselves we make better choices. We want to take care of ourselves, and our reasons for eating changes. We stop searching for comfort from our food and start eating foods that nourish our body, mind & soul completely. Foods like organic greens, vegetables, fruits, legumes and whole grains. The need to muscle our willpower into the equation to make us eat these foods disappears, simply because we have a more effective strategy for dealing with our emotions. A strategy that make us feel more in control, safer, freer and more deeply nourished than we have felt in a long time. And the funny thing is that only a small percentage of the population is applying this common sense approach. By maintaining their weight loss naturally, having more laughs, enjoying the benefits of having more energy all while living a less stressful and more enjoyable life! Simply because they feel good about themselves and make choices that nourish & up-lift them instead of depending on willpower and self control.

I said it a moment ago and I'll say it again because it's that important: when we feel good about ourselves, we naturally embark on a healthier lifestyle and make more nourishing choices in all areas of our lives. Choices that are our priority because they empower us, nurture us and enable us to thrive and enjoy life. There simply is no need for "willpower" anymore.

As women, for most of our lives, we've been taught that we need to take care of others before we take care of ourselves. We need to put the group before the individual and that is commendable; but you can't give from an empty vessel. Even in an airplane, we are instructed to give oxygen to ourselves first, before we give it to our children so we can assist them better and keep them safe! If we have nothing of substance to offer those who mean so much to us, then no one benefits.

As women, we are caregivers by nature. We're loving, nurturing and will make huge sacrifices to make others happy. This is a fabulous quality. Yet I often wonder what the world would be like if more women were as nurturing to themselves, as they are to the others in their lives. I wonder how many relationships would improve if more women were taught to have more self assurance and to take care of nourishing themselves first, before giving their time and energy to those they love. I wonder how it would affect our young girls as they grow up in the world and how they would develop into adults. Would they be more empowered with a more positive role model, someone who appreciates their unique qualities, and truly believes that they can do anything they set their minds to do that is of great value to them, instead of being someone who was never happy with what they have or how they look, constantly cycling though different diets (*and kids do pick up on everything we say and do*), only motivated by keeping up appearances of importance and health. I wonder how many people in the world would be less stressed, healthier, happier and more genuinely nourished simply because they made choices that were a priority to them. Choices that allowed them to thrive, instead of just survive.

Self-care really is at the core of managing stress and mindless emotional eating, it has very little to do with willpower. Without making the time to listen to our needs and trust our inner voice, we will sabotage our success each and every time. If you've ridden the never ending roller coaster of eating healthy, eating poorly, eating healthy, eating poorly, or my other favorite; starving, binging, starving, binging, and struggled to figure out why you were so moody, so tired, so depressed and just can't seem to lose that muffin top, you know what I'm talking about.

## <u>Take A Mindful Moment:</u>
*(Part 1)*

1. On a piece of paper write down all the things you enjoy doing; ways you take care of yourself and show yourself love, care and nurturing. This could be a long, soak in the tub with a book, it could be getting your toes done, it could be cuddling up with a pet or that some special, or going to a yoga class. Whatever makes you feel good.

2. Now write the specific benefits you experience physically, mentally and emotionally. Use as many adjectives as you can to really get to the heart of what makes these activities so rewarding for you.

3. Write out a typical daily schedule and color code your activities, making sure that you include time in there to nurture yourself. Example: blue-work, red-kids activities, green-household chores, pink-me time.

*Make time for yourself.* Add your needs into your daily schedule. Make your needs (what makes you feel most nourished) a priority and watch how willpower takes a back seat.

## Take A Mindful Moment:
*(Part 2)*

Now that you've started including more time for yourself to do activities that nurture you, we can begin to become more aware of what your priorities are. What motives you to take action?

1.  On a piece of paper, make note of what is important to you in your life. Who is important to you? What lifestyle you cherish? What type of attitude do you admire and aspire to ….

2.  Now imagine what it would be like if all your choices were made when weighed against this marker. How would your choices be different? What changes in your thoughts do you think would occur?

3.  For the next 10 days every decision you make will be made based on these priorities. So if a priority for you is to have less stress, and more balance, start telling people that you have too much on your plate and you just are not able to volunteer for that activity; or start clearing away the excess clutter in your environment. This could mean cleaning up & organizing your house to just taking some time away from toxic relationships.

**PS:** *Continue to be tuning into your tastes & emotions. Before you know it, this skill will become second nature and you will start creating a better relationship with your cravings.*

# COACHING SESSION 3:
## *Listening For Triggers*

How did you do as you were writing down all the ways, you take care of yourself and show yourself love, care and nurturing?

Did you make choices that were based on your priorities for 10 days?

Will I need to check up on you again?

No?

Good.

The main purpose of this book, is to give you the opportunity to experiment with new concepts as you learn them, just as I do with my coaching clients. So if you're actually playing with these Mindful Moments, keep it up! You may be unraveling parts of yourself that have been closed up for far too long…

Earlier we discussed the definition of cravings as "An intense, urgent, or abnormal desire or longing to consume something". Unfortunately, many of us view our cravings as a sign of weakness or something that is disconnected and separated from ourselves. Like some sort of outside invader that we need to fight or do battle with. And this makes me sad, because cravings are really just the body/mind's way of telling us that it needs better nourishment for balance & improved performance. While skipping meals like breakfast or lunch may seem like a good idea when we're stressed, we need to remember the results of those actions afterwards. It's important to remember how anxious we may tend to get when we don't eat, how hard it gets to concentrate, and how ravenous we'll get later in the day because we're starving! And keep in mind that when we do finally eat after starving ourselves, it's usually food we end up feeling remorseful & guilty for eating or we start mindlessly bingeing on whatever is in arm's reach.

What would happen if, instead of skipping that meal and depriving ourselves of what we need, we paused for a moment, then really listened to what our body is crying out for so we could better understand it? How would we tell the difference between a cry for genuine nourishment and a good old-fashioned temper tantrum (otherwise known as an intense craving)?

Well, it comes down to being aware of our unique needs, which includes being able to listen to (and trust) those subtle clues we tend to push aside or stuff down with food. For our purposes here, we'll simplify it and separate the two different types of cravings. This way it will be easier to tune in to our natural instincts, and trust what bubbles up to the surface. After helping a variety of women from all over the country learn how to trust their intuition again, I have to share with you that you really do know a lot more than you may be giving yourself credit for. So trust that subtle, quiet voice within. She really loves you.

Think of it like this:

Imagine you're in a store and, while shopping, you can hear some child screaming at the top of their lungs, doing their best to stress out their poor mother. They may embarrass her so much that she gives in to their demands, no matter what they are. And if not, the child gets louder and louder, even going so far as to kick and flail about, causing such a fuss that their stressed-out, tired mother ends up giving in, only because she knows once she does, the chaos will stop for a little while, and she can go about her shopping with a few moments of sanity.

That, my friend, is a temper-tantrum craving, or what I call our "Inner Spoiled Brat". That's an example of what "an intense, urgent, or abnormal desire or longing to consume something" can be like. Can you see the parallel?

When was the last time you gave into your Inner Spoiled Brat?

Giving into a voracious craving is no different from a mother giving into her screaming child. No matter how much we may pacify the temper-tantrum for the moment, it only becomes more intense later, and tends to become more demanding as it grows.

On the flip side, imagine a mother who takes the time to understand her child's unique needs and prepares for them. She is aware of her child's temperament, personal schedule and is prepared with nourishing foods, activities or both, before she goes out to run errands to ensure they both have an enjoyable experience. She listens and communicates in a clear, positive way while checking in with her child periodically, and is able to prevent a possible breakdown by taking these actions. Everyone is happy; everyone is content, and both of them are able to go about their day with a genuine smile on their face. No matter what may pop up along the way.

When we listen to, and are aware of, the subtle messages our body shares with us (what I call our "Inner Nutrition Guru"), our cravings become more manageable like the "Balanced Child" in this example, who can go shopping without stressing out her mother.

Now I ask you, which scenario would you rather go through day in and day out?

What do you believe could trigger our cravings ?

The answer…a number of things. Like what we see, smell, touch, read about or hear someone talking about. These are what I call "sensory cravings" and they're things we didn't want or crave, until they were brought to our attention through one of our five senses. Which then triggers a memory, a feeling or an emotion that amy be happy, soothing or comforting. When we're overwhelmed, stressed-out or struggling with a variety of challenges in our lives, we naturally want to be comforted and regain our balance. So those triggered foods become appealing.

Here's how I discovered this... A couple of weeks ago I was driving down the road when all of a sudden I could smell hamburgers cooking from a local restaurant as I drove by. Now for those of you who don't know, I've stopped eating cow's meat for many years now. Just the idea, literally turns my stomach. This is why I was so incredibly surprised when the smell of these burgers cooking made me crave, actually, crave one! Then I imagined what it would be like to actually be eating that burger. I checked in with myself to find out if giving in to this sudden craving would nourish and satisfy me or make me feel sick. I imagined what it would look like and feel like in my hands as I was holding it. I imagined what it would taste like as it touched my tongue on the first bite, the texture in my mouth, what it would taste like as I continued chewing...and I couldn't go any further. I was starting to feel like I was going to puke right there in the car. Then I asked myself *why* I wanted the burger in the first place. I wanted to know what triggered it. Then it hit me like a flash of lightening. It was the distinctive smell of those specific burgers cooking.

Ok, now, I've smelled burgers cooking, and never before had it ever had the same affect on me. There was something about the unique smell of those particular burgers wafting throughout the air, that I had to have. So before I mindlessly grabbed a burger, I wondered, what was it that I was *really* craving, because I knew that it certainly wasn't what I was smelling.

Slowly it came to me. That particular smell reminded me of the days when I was little. Back to the days when my dad would grill burgers, with me as his little assistant, in the backyard, in the middle of the winter, with the snow falling down on us. I remembered putting my little feet in his big boots, which went all the way up to my hips, just to go outside and help him. I remembered him smiling down at me while snow dusted his hair, teaching me about the "right" way to cook a burger. It was one of the rare, warm and loving memories I had of a time I got to bond with my dad; just me and him. THAT was what I was craving… the emotional connection I had with him at that time. And the smell triggered my memory of feeling safe, loved and happy. So instead of getting the burger, I called my dad. We had a really nice conversation, and when the call was done, I gave myself a bid hug pretending that it was him hugging me. And just like that, my craving was satisfied.

Years ago, I never would have been able to do that. Why? Well, to be honest I didn't know it was an option! I didn't know that cravings could be for something other than food! And not only did I not know that I could satisfy my cravings this way, but at that point in my life I hadn't trusted myself enough to go through the process of figuring out what I really needed. It took my deep desire for something different than what I had and small consistent, mindful actions to establish a new relationship between me, my Inner Nutrition Guru and my triggers. Once it was in place though, I began to wonder where it had been all my life! I suddenly had the clarity, the confidence and the control over my outcomes that I never had before. It was exhilarating! And this new relationship was one I had decided right then and there I was going to cherish, because I was a keeper.

Our relationships are important. With the people, we share our lives with, sure, but most importantly with ourselves first. I mean how can we ask someone to give us something we aren't willing to give to ourselves?

Whenever I begin a new relationship with a woman I'll be working with, I'll ask her, "How often do you trust your instincts?" Which is often met with a long stare at me, as if I was speaking another language. Then I ask it another way, "How often do you listen to and trust your quiet inner voice or your intuition to make decisions that benefit you?" Which is then met with a quick eye-opening of understanding, followed by a drooping of shoulders or a dropping of the head followed by a quiet response of, "Not very often". So I'll ask, "Why not? What's stopping you?" and gradually, throughout our conversation, she begins to gain a greater awareness of the wisdom she already possesses. and over a couple of sessions, positive self-awareness, self-respect and self-compassion take root.

Each one of us makes the choice to eat for our own personal reasons. Maybe it's for escape, maybe it's for comfort, maybe it's because something triggers you to eat.

Was food really, what you were craving, or was it something else? And who were you indulging, your Inner Spoiled Brat or Inner Nutrition Guru?

I've shared a bit of what I've learned with you. Now you get to make some personal discoveries of your own...

## Take a Mindful Moment:

Why are you eating? What triggered you to eat? Before you actually do this exercise, I'd like you to read the whole thing first. The goal is to help you connect with your inner wisdom, or what I call your "Inner Nutrition Guru". By doing this, you will be able to better understand the difference between your "spoiled brat" screaming for something in the moment, and a true desire for nourishment.

Cravings are simply the body's way of communicating what it needs. When we understand our body's language, we begin to work with our cravings rather than battling against them. Creating a balanced relationship, where we get to have pleasure, be truly satiated and nourished, instead of suffering with guilt, shame or disappointment.

Remember that each one of us has a relationship with ourselves as well as with our food, and our food has a place in every aspect of our lives. Food can be our genuine friend, instead of our frienemy. Just like any relationship, our relationship with food takes a little awareness, careful listening, thoughtfulness, flexibility and lots of love. The more we are mindfully aware of our unique needs, consistently listening to and trusting our Inner Nutrition Guru, the better we understand those needs and how to meet them in a way that empowers us. This makes us more confident when making choices that satisfy us in every area of our lives. Subsequently, we effectively reduce cravings almost overnight.

*Just follow along....*

As you sit and read this, focus in on your breathing. Notice how the inhalation is cool as it comes into your body, and the exhalation is warm as the air leaves your body. Simply follow your breath going in and out for a few moments. Now, you may notice that your breath in and breath out is moving rhythmically. Each breath is rising and falling at a pace just right for you, with very little effort. Maybe it's feeling a bit soothing, even relaxing.

Focus your attention now on where you feel most relaxed in your body. Allow that feeling to flow into your entire being, from your head to your toes, as if it is liquid gently flowing over each area, allowing it to totally relax. Wherever you find yourself knotted up, each breath out loosens up its grip, and makes space for relaxation, comfort and peace. Your breath may now be a bit deeper and more relaxed, enabling your whole body, including your mind, to simply let go.

As you drift away in this peaceful space, ask your inner self what it is that would truly nourish you. What is it you need? The answer may come to you in a picture, a word or a feeling allowing your initial natural answer to easily flow into your awareness thus freeing you of any judgment, expectations or doubt.

Imagine your body as your baby. When the baby cries, how are you caring for it? What are the subtle cries and clues your body is giving you for attention and to fill the void you're experiencing? Again, it comes to you in an image, maybe it comes from a voice within your mind, and maybe it's a feeling or a taste. The answer may not even be food. It could be something else entirely.

Continue to breathe into your belly button, as you relax even further. Now however your relaxation has more clarity. You feel more refreshed, and know what you need.

Go ahead and take the actions that nourish your heart, mind and soul.

Clearly listening to the body/mind helps us better understand what is most nourishing to us every moment of the day and is great for preventing cravings from coming on intensely and in a toxic way.

I suggest for the next 7 days keeping a journal to keep track of the messages your Inner Nutrition Guru gives you, and what you actually choose. Keeping track of what happens when you listen to your body versus when you listen to your critical, educated mind can heighten your awareness to what is actually going on (instead of what we think we remember, which is not always so accurate) and help you begin to make more nourishing choices.

*P.S. Oh, by-the-way....*

**Habitual dieters tend to ignore their baby**, and typically only listen to the criticizing mental chatter going on instead. It's a constant nagging voice that is berating, abusing and criticizing them all day long. After a while not only do they not realize it's there, it is actually a comfort because it's what they know. So there is reluctance to change it from the inside out, instead of what they are typically doing, which is trying to change from the outside in with little long lasting results.

If most of us had a friend who spoke to us in such a negative way all the time, they would no longer be a friend. So why do we allow such talk to go on in our own head when we talk to ourselves?

This only teaches us not to trust ourselves. We need to trust ourselves if we are ever going to prevent any future cravings from getting the better of us.

By taking action to listen to our baby, inner wisdom, inner nutrition guru or whatever you want to call it (maybe you want to go with Sally), we honor our unique needs. We embrace ourselves for the individual that we are, and nourish ourselves with what we need, instead of what we are told we should want. We stop denying ourselves what we crave the most-love, compassion, a sense of worth, self-love and self-respect.

When we consciously choose foods that help the baby stop crying we reduce cravings, mood swings and depression. We begin to better understand our unique needs physically, mentally, emotionally & spiritually in a way that is truly enriching and empowering.

# COACHING SESSION 4:

*Wholistic Nutrition-*
*Feeding the Mind, Body & Soul*

Recently I had a very interesting conversation with a new client of mine, I'll call her Annie (although it's not her real name). After a little bit of conversation, Annie shared with me that she just couldn't trust herself around food. She believed she was the victim of her emotions and food was her only savior. Whenever she felt overwhelmed and emotions started to overpower her, she would run to her comfort food and let it have control of the situation so she could feel better. It was the only thing she believed she could count on when she felt that way. The trouble was, she constantly found herself mindlessly over-indulging and drowning her sorrows in her food, then mentally berating herself afterwards for eating too much, yet again. She would feel so horrible inside, she would often breakdown and cry, because she felt like "such a loser" wondering how other people seemed to manage to eat without having a problem like this. After carefully listening to her story, I asked her to explain in more detail, where exactly in her life she felt the most overwhelmed or out of control. She paused and thought about it for a moment, then told me she felt the most stressed and overwhelmed when she was trying to balance her work responsibilities and her home life responsibilities. She felt she didn't have a moment to herself even to just go to the bathroom. It was if she was drowning under the load of her commitments to other people. She just wanted some breathing room.

I continued to listen carefully as she continued, then asked her another question. I wanted to know, how she knew specifically, she was beginning to feel overwhelmed with stress filled emotions. Was something she felt, a voice she heard in her head, or maybe something she saw in her minds eye or in front of her (like a pile of laundry)? Again she paused. She thought and thought, until she finally told me that she knew she was overwhelmed, when everything looked like chaos to her. Everywhere she looked, at home and at work, even as she drove in her car, all she saw was chaos. Things that needed to be put in their places, organized and made tidy which would set her off. She would start to feel tight in her shoulders, her breathing would be faster and her stomach would get in knots. That's when she would reach for the comfort food. She wanted the knots in her stomach to unravel, and in the past she thought it had always worked for her. Now she wasn't so sure.

After hearing this, I wanted to get a better understanding of her perspective of food, and the role it played in her life. When I asked her what food was, she paused for a moment and looked at me strangely. As if to say, "Are you not from this planet?" But after a couple of beats, she proceeded to list all sorts of foods you would find in a grocery store, such as grapes, eggs, milk and so on, then explained that food was what we ate for breakfast, lunch and dinner. It gave us energy to do the things we wanted to do and could make us fat if we ate too much. I could tell she thought I was nuts, because when she was finished, she again looked at me strangely. After all, wasn't I supposed to know what food was? I am the professional after all, and she was coming to me for help. I continued on and asked her if she ever heard of the phrase, "Food for Thought". She paused again and assured me she had heard the phrase before. Next, I asked her if she ever had to "digest" some information before she made a decision, she said yes. Then I asked her my final question; if she could remember ever having such a good time doing something a bit stressful but fun, like going on a roller coaster or taking a trip, that she didn't think about her comfort foods. She thought about it for a moment then told me she had. So I explained to her that everything I just mentioned are all examples of "food" through the eyes of Wholistic Nutrition*.

*(If you are wondering why I spell the word <u>W</u>holistic instead of <u>H</u>olistic, it's because I personally dislike the word being spelled with an H. To me that spelling leaves a Hole in the true meaning of what Wholistic health is all about. It seems to have become a simple marketing tool many use without an understanding how the whole interconnected web of thoughts, emotions & energy affect our entire well-being physically, mentally, emotionally & spiritually. That is it goes far beyond the physical, and deeper than any marketing tactic.)

From a <u>w</u>holistic perspective, food is much more than just a bunch of individual vitamins, nutrients or calories. In fact, what we've been taught about nutrition is really only the introduction to a much bigger story. A story that includes a multi-faceted understanding of true nourishment physically, mentally, emotionally and yes, even spiritually. A story that takes us on a never ending journey of awakening and awareness, struggle and achievement, curiosity and love. A story that can enrich our very soul.

According to its definition, food is anything we take in to the body to help maintain life and help us grow. And since science can now verify that there is no separation between the body & mind, that they do indeed act interchangeably, it's time to upgrade our understanding of food and its impact on our lives as well.

Food includes everything from our thoughts, our beliefs, relationships & social lives, to our career & finances. It impacts the total well-being of our body/mind, as well as our quality of our lives. It incorporates our home environment & home cooking, our physical activities, spirituality and creativity, as well as the very substances we put into our mouths every day. By creating balance in each individual aspect of our lives, and blending them with an awareness of the physical foods we eat (foods that are best suited to our unique needs), we begin to develop a more optimally nourishing life, and enjoy all the benefits of genuine whole health.

From the viewpoint of wholistic nutrition, we understand that our food is much more than just the consumable products we take in, digest and absorb through our mouths. We understand that food goes beyond our simple notion of fats, proteins, carbohydrates, vitamins, minerals, calories so on. We know that we can be truly nourished by what we take in through our mind as well as our body. We're aware that what we choose to think, and say to ourselves can impact our ability to experience true nourishment. Because if we're constantly focused on what is wrong or lacking with ourselves or our lives, as well as what's wrong with other people, we create a subtle level of malnourishment that leaves us craving more satisfaction. We're looking for the rest of what we're missing to complete us and make us whole. And it can be as simple as weighing our options and asking ourselves, "How does this nourish me physically, mentally or spiritually?" before making a decision. Even if that decision is what to eat.

When we're only focused on our limitations, it's as if we're sitting in a cave, with a little bit of light, and all we can see are the rocks around us. We miss out on the fact that we're actually sitting in a cave filled with diamonds. When we're not focused on nourishing our whole selves physically, mentally, emotionally & spiritually, we're missing out on the best part of our food and our life.

We can choose to make more uplifting, centering and empowering decisions or we can do exactly what we've always been doing and get the same toxic, self deprived, self defeating results over and over again.

And at the end of the day, when we lay our heads on the pillow, reflecting on our lives, we begin to realize…Just because we ate the latest super-foods, watched our calorie intake, and went to the gym, it doesn't mean we're truly nourished. There's something still lacking; A part of the puzzle that's missing.

We're taught to only focus on only one aspect of nutrition; physical health. It's what we read about, hear about and is advertised in every possible place imaginable. Our governmental "Choose My Plate" guidelines suggest proteins, grains, vegetables and fruits all shown proportionally on a plate with a glass of milk on the side. Which honestly, is better than it was in the past, but where's the water? A human being is made up of almost 85% water. Our brain depends on water to function properly. Without it we become fatigued, and lose our ability to have clear, focused thinking. And very few nutrition articles actually tell us <u>how</u> we are to know which foods are right for us as individuals versus the masses. When we look at nutrition from a wholistic nutrition perspective, every person has unique nutritional needs based on their personal chemical make-up, their body type, their heredity and more. If those in power truly want us to be healthy, they need to teach the public how to be more aware of all aspects of nutrition, and not just a small aspect of it. They need to teach people how to have a better understanding of how various foods affect them (which is what I do in my classes, groups and workshops) and stop allowing lobby groups to determine our source of information and education.

One of the greatest lessons I've learned over the years, is that nourishment supersedes nutrition. We can eat all the nutritious foods we want, however, if we're feeling emotionally overwhelmed, stressed-out or lacking in any other area of our lives, what we eat and its nutrient content, won't matter. It will all end up in the toilet, instead of getting to our cells and nourishing us. We instinctively know that we need the other half of the story for optimal nourishment, for us to be complete.

When we have a greater awareness and better understanding of our unique needs, then take loving and compassionate actions to fill those needs, we create more balance in every area of our lives. And we thrive. The funny thing is, that many times our unique needs are easily satisfied by one of Life's Foods, instead of the physical foods we been limited to be aware of.

Life's Foods take our understanding of food to a whole new level. Because we are nourished physically, mentally, emotionally & spiritually with things that go far beyond what we put on our plates or in our cups. Remember, food is everything from our beliefs & thoughts, to our satisfaction in our relationship & career. It's our home environment & home cooking, our physical activities, spirituality and creativity. When we experience genuine nourishment, fulfillment and enjoyment in any and all of these areas, they enrich our lives and make the physical food we eat that much more effective for us, because they actually are all forms of food.

Remember the last time you were totally consumed with a hobby or a project you enjoyed and thoughts of eating never entered your mind. Think back to what it was like as a child to play with such intensity and joy, that all you could focus on was what you were playing because it was so much fun. In fact, you had such a good time, that when you were called in for dinner, and the street lamps were turned on, it barely even registered that your mom was calling for you. These are just two examples of how we receive nourishment from Life's Foods. If you're a runner you may have experienced it in the "high" you get when you run, as a yoga practitioner you have most likely felt it as you finished your flow and relaxed in savasana. You may get it when you write, or paint or play with clay. It can be so many little things, as well as the big moments, we take part in throughout our daily lives.

We may feel satisfied in our work when we are contributing to the lives of others in a positive way, feeling totally nourished with our career choice. Sure, we may have frustrating days, it's part of the job. Yet we're able to work through them more easily because our job satisfies and completes us on a deeper level than just for the money. After long day of work, when walk into a home that is decorated in a way that is welcoming, relaxing and even tidy, it makes us feel as if we can freely let go of the tension we may have been holding on to, allowing us to feel nourished in that space. Our relationship with family members can also play a role in our level of nourishment, as can the relationship we have with ourselves.

The relationship we have with ourselves through our inner talk, whether it is filled with compassion, understanding and love or with loathing, hatred and judgment, can often determine how we will relate to others in our lives. If our intimate relationship with ourselves is negative, very few relationships will ever be able to satisfy us the way we most deeply desire. We will constantly be looking for that piece of the puzzle that won't be there until we put it in place. Sure others may be able to nourish us with a hug when we are down, a shoulder to lean on when we need someone to talk to, make us laugh until we think we're going to pee, or relate to us in a way that no other person can, simply because they just "get" us. However, it's the relationship we have with ourselves, once balanced and filled with love & self-awareness, that helps us see the true role people play in our lives; whether they are toxic and prevent us from being true to ourselves or genuinely nourishing and accepting, lifting us up and enabling us to be the best version of ourselves.

Because just like junk food, if a friendship is not nourishing you, it's harming you. And that relationship is a part of your Life's Foods and contributes to your total well-being.

Everything is made up of energy, just ask your local quantum physicist; and that includes our food too. Our physical food has a life of its own, which includes the animals we eat, as well as the plants and grains. Each one carries its own unique rhythms of energy that we take into ourselves as we eat and digest it. And this is true of the energy we put into our food as we are preparing it as well.

Many of us rush around making our breakfast or lunch in the morning before work feeling totally stressed. Then when we finally sit down to eat, we are not only digesting the food we prepared, we're also digesting those stressed-out, negative feelings, making them more powerful; deeply embedding them into each and every one of our cells. And our body believes what we tell it.

On the other hand, if we show genuine gratitude for our food as we prepare it, and are excited about the smells, the colors and anticipate how good it will taste before we eat it, we absorb all the nutrients of that food, along with the blessings of gratitude and love, creating a truly nourishing meal and an opportunity for optimal digestion.

Without beating you over the head with this information, I think you get the idea by now.

*So now it's your turn...*

# Take a Mindful Moment:

Wholistic nutrition goes far beyond just what we put in our mouths, it's a bigger understanding of what true nourishment really is and how it affects every part of us; impacting our neurology, our biology, our chemistry and so much more.

So where are you nourished and where could you use a bit more attention?

I suggest going through this exercise at least once a week for 4 weeks before going to the next coaching session, to get a better handle of how your Life's Foods affect you on a daily basis. We are constantly changing and evolving, so you may want to use this as your personal "check-in" meter. I found it particularly helpful when I first started in creating a greater awareness of my personal needs. That awareness gave me the insight I needed to create more balance in my life by getting rid of the things ( *yes, including relationships*) that we're toxic to me and including more of the things that helped be flourish.

On a separate piece of paper, make a large circle. Now divide the circle into 12 pie wedges so you can fit in a spot for each area of your whole health.

Those areas are: *(next page)*

Begin by asking yourself "Am I being nourished?" when you review each area. And rate it 1 (lowest) to 10 (highest) in your head, then put it on the chart. For example, if you feel you are totally satisfied and fulfilled in your career, give it a 10. However, if you feel it is lacking in sooo many ways, and potentially toxic for you give it a 2 or a 1. If it falls somewhere in between, meaning you enjoy it but things could be better, give it a 4, 5 or 6.

| Self Worth | Home Cooking | Education |
| --- | --- | --- |
| Relationships | Home Environment | Career |
| Social Life | Whole Foods | Finances |
| Physical Activity | Creativity | Spirituality |

Now color in the wedges-Red for anything that is a 3 or less, Yellow for anything 4-6, and Green for 7-10.

After doing this exercise, observe what you have colored in. Where are you malnourished and need more attention? Where do you thrive and experience joy & nourishment?

What single thought or action step can you take to bring you closer to wholeness and balance?

Remember to be true to yourself. What would genuinely nourish you in each of these areas if you had a magic wand and could have your wish granted? Write down what you would see, hear and feel on a typical day.

You have permission to dream big and in technicolor!

# COACHING SESSION 5:
*Your Stress Monster & You*

Got Stress? How many times have you suddenly realized that you've overextended yourself, and are now being pulled in all different directions, stretched to your limits like a piece of taffy? Have you ever eaten while feeling that way? Who hasn't, right?

Our modern lifestyles have us on this never-ending hamster wheel. We wake up after a restless sleep filled with worries, fears and anxieties, and get out of bed totally groggy, knowing we need to hurry because we overslept again. We know we have to eat, so after getting our morning coffee started, showering, blow-drying our hair, putting on make-up and figuring out what to wear that actually fits, we grab something to shove in our mouths and rush out the door. Does that sound familiar?

While at work, we might be behind on a deadline, or handed a new pile of work, adding to the never ending pile we already have. We become overwhelmed with everything that needs to get done in what seems to be a short amount of time. At some point we may notice we're craving something or simply need a distraction from all the chaos. So we grab something out of the vending machine, or grab a remaining pastry from the kitchen, and head back to work with our food in our mouths. On the way home from work, we may suddenly realize how hungry we are because we've barely eaten during the day. So we stop off at one of our favorite drive-thrus and get something to eat before we even make it home. Once we get home, there's still no time to put our feet up, chill out and simply breathe. We need to check the kids homework, make dinner and maybe even take the kids to their extracurricular activities. So as the kids do their homework, we throw something together, put it on the table, rush through our meals and away we go. Many times barely noticing what we're putting into our mouths, let alone what our food tastes like-unless it tastes absolutely disgusting or exceptionally tasty.

In essence, our lives have become a slave to the clock and in turn, we've become immersed in stress or as it's now called 'Super-Stress'. We're "on-call" 24/7 to our texts, email, social media, cell phones, tablets, laptops and more. What's even more surprising, is that the entertainment so many of us depend on to help us relax and de-stress at the end of a challenging day, actually adds to our stress and anxieties! In a 2012 article written in Psychology Today, a study was done to find out how all the increasing negative sensationalized news actually affects us. They discovered that people's worries become worse and anxieties higher with more negative news broadcasts being shown. "Reality" TV is easy to get drawn into with all its over the top drama, diva antics and rags to riches stories. However, a small handful of studies now show us that these shows can actually do some damage to our ability in handling our real life stress. Even watching any of the various crime dramas or medical shows that seem real, can impact our ability to decompress in our own lives and to replenish our self healing resources. And because we're constantly plugged in and on the go, we're often sitting in front of the TV and eating during any of these high stress shows, or connected to any of our numerous electronic devices as we have a meal.

Maybe this will blow you mind the way it blew mine: with all this stressful stimulation and unrest, just eating something deemed "healthy" by the experts, is not really going to make that much of a difference; because if you're eating while stressed, a majority of those nutrients are going straight into the toilet and not getting where they will do you any good. More about that in a bit, I promise.

OK-pause.

Breathe…. into your belly. Breathe….in…Breathe…out…

Instead of letting our minds wander off as we start thinking about what needs to get done in our lives, as stress begins to pile up, let's pause for a moment and take a nice deep breath into our belly buttons……

Feel the oxygen flow into your nose, down into your diaphragm, gently expanding your belly, easily and effortlessly, free of any force or trying to; simply being with the breath. And hold for the count of four, three, two, one.

Now with a deep sigh, let it out, releasing all the tension from your shoulders, your back, and your belly simply go free. Slowly, roll you head around for a moment. Notice where you feel lighter, more airy and feel more free…

Repeat this one more time…Inhale into your diaphragm, feeling cooling, refreshing air enter into your nose…and Exhale and let go of all the tension from your mind, let your lips and your jaw natural part, let your tongue feel slack, now your throat, your shoulders and your belly. Just let it all go…every muscle, bone and tight spot opening up and becoming light and airy. Maybe you even feel like you could totally float now.

Feel a bit better? OK, now we can continue feeling a bit more relaxed. And I've been told we learn more when we're relaxed, so let's continue.

We experience stress everyday, yet we know very little about this monster that seems to take over our lives. The key to taming and controlling our personal stress monster is to understand what makes it tick, what activates it within us and to ultimately create a better relationship with it, so we can manipulate it in a way that works for us, instead of allowing the stress monster to make us its victim.

Let's begin by understanding the three stages of stress. I promise, this will not be one of those boring science lessons. Instead, it's simply some background information that will help you better understand the creature you'll be working with; no different from an introduction to someone at a party I wanted you to meet or to a new colleague at work. I want you to have all the tools you need for a successful, positive relationship. And as with any healthy relationship, it depends on our full attention, our awareness and love. This helps us get out of our own way, more easily creating a life of less fear, and filling it instead with more self confidence and peace of mind.

## Stress typically comes on in three stages:

*The first is called the alarm stage,* which is when our adrenal glands are triggered to kick into action and release a surge of energy so we can either fight, freeze or run like hell. Our heart rate increases, blood flow surges, hearing and eyesight temporarily becomes a bit sharper, muscles tense and activate, our blood sugar rises as our liver releases stored sugars into our bloodstream, and we are primed for action.

*The second stage is known as the resistance stage.* This usually activates when the alarm stage wasn't just a passing thing, such as when we have a close call with another car as we're driving down the road. In that case, our stress would be a fleeting thing, because it happened and was resolved quickly. Resistance stage stress hangs out for a while, causing our body/mind to prepare for a longer fight. The adrenal glands begin to draw on any nutritional reserves we may have, to give us longer lasting energy so we can make it through whatever may be our stressful event.

This may last for a little while, but as soon as those reserves are used up, cell-damaging free radicals begin to form in larger and larger numbers. Leaving us exhausted, with a weaker immune system, poor digestion, poor brain function and in a bad mood, craving things we would never eat if we were stronger & healthier. Here's an additional tidbit of information for you, during this stage the collagen & elasticity in our skin also begins to break down more quickly, creating more wrinkles and fine lines due to free radical damage. So if you have a hard time wrapping your mind around the health aspects of stress, it may be more motivating for you to reduce your stress if it means that it also affects your youthful appearance.

*The third stage is Exhaustive Stress.* This is where 'Super-Stress' lives, and unfortunately, where most of us who are living the typical American lifestyle are right now. During this stage, stress in unrelenting. All of the reserves the adrenal glands draw from are depleted. But they don't know that. They just keep on doing what they do naturally, and release the hormones adrenaline, noradrenalin and cortisol in a futile attempt to help us deal with our stress better. As adrenal exhaustion becomes more prominent, all of our organ systems begin to experience the burden as well, and that often leads to imbalances within the body such as hypoglycemia, low sex drive, poor immune function, high blood pressure, anxiety, depression and more. The crazy thing is that because we have access to so many convenient food-like substances, we think we are helping ourselves by putting those "enriched" foods into our bodies. The truth is that by doing this, we're actually depleting our reserve storehouse before stress even has a chance to make its mark. Because in order for the body to metabolize those refined, sugary "enriched" foods, it needs to take stored-up nutrients from our body to do it. Which leaves even less resources available for our adrenals when we need them most.

I think of it like a bank. When the bank account is full and abundant, we can pay bills, go shopping and really enjoy ourselves. However when the account is low, and we depend on credit cards to continue the good times, instead of laying low and just taking it easy, we're creating more debt and more stress, by spending money we don't actually have. Imagine what it would be like if that was how you lived your life and you went to get groceries, then suddenly realized all your credit cards and your bank account was maxed out? Would it leave you feeling depressed, depleted and stressed out? I imagine so...

Stress is defined as "any real or imagined threat and our response to that threat". Today's fast-paced lifestyle attacks our nervous system constantly and what I find incredibly interesting is that most of our modern day stress is the creation of our own minds, or how we perceive things be. Yet our nervous systems can't tell the difference between a real, or a vividly imagined threat. No matter where it comes from, it will still react the same way.

Pause for a moment, wherever you are right now, and think of something that's been stressing you out over the last couple of days. Seriously, do this now. Recall all the details of that specific reason or event causing you to worry, to become anxious or fearful. As it comes to the surface of your memory, and becomes more real to you in your mind right now, check in with your breathing. Maybe you've noticed that its gotten a bit faster, maybe it's coming from your chest instead of your belly, and is more shallow. Maybe your heart is beating a bit faster and you're experiencing some discomfort in your stomach, the muscles in your shoulders may have gotten tighter, and you find you're clenching your jaw. The effects of this memory are very real, yet there was no real physical threat at this moment. The threat was all in your mind.

This may be rather eye opening. Because even if we can just imagine suffering in some way, our adrenal glands release the same stress chemicals to fight, freeze or run away. Although this reaction would be incredibly helpful during an actual threat, we tend to use up these natural super powers of sharper thinking, seeing and hearing with a jolt to our muscle strength, as well as our nutrient supply, on stressful thoughts we can neither fight nor run away from in that moment. We tend to become so tangled up in negative thinking, that we stay stuck in it, until we decide to cut ourselves loose by focusing on what is real and true in this moment right now. Over time, as we begin to reach the exhaustive stage, those stress chemicals, which are still being released, become toxic and cause a host of imbalances within our body/mind.

*Check it out....*

Acid Reflux

Digestive Disturbances

Low Sex Drive

Rapid Heartbeat

Headache

Rapid Breathing

Acne

Psoriasis or Eczema

Low Blood Sugar

Urinary Tract Infections

Easily Susceptible to Infections

A Stiff Neck With Tight Shoulders

An Upset Stomach, Nausea, or Diarrhea

Back Pain

Arthritis

Osteoporosis

Chronic Pain

Candidiasis

Weight Gain

## How many of those could you check off?

And do you know what trigger's your stress? Most times our triggers can be put into the category of either environmental, social, physical, or mental/emotional.

As you go through your day, you may want to take a mindful moment to check in with yourself so you can uncover your personal triggers, how it affects you, as well as what the most effective remedy is to help you stop stress from overwhelming you.

## Sources of Stress:

<u>Environmental</u>

noise

air pollution

plant pollens

weather

traffic

<u>Social</u>

large gatherings

deadlines

financial

job interviews or new job

time management

loss of a loved one

personality conflicts

Physical

lack of physical activity or too much

hormonal imbalance

rapid growth in adolescence

aging

injuries

sickness

malnutrition

dehydration

physical threat


Mental/Emotional

worry

anxiety

guilt

boredom

fear

frustration

self-image

internal perception of situation

recalling similar past experience

a need to control everything/everyone


**Any of these sources of stress can trigger us to seek out comfort.** Unfortunately though, many of us gravitate to food when feeling overwhelmed, since it's so easily available and we have the belief that we can control it when it seems we can control nothing else.

Before we go any further though, let's check in with ourselves to take a mindful moment.

## Take a Mindful Moment:

I'm pretty sure you can tell when you're stressed once you've reached the exhaustive stage. But are you aware of how stress effects you during the other stages? You know, before it overtakes your very life? Do you know how to turn off your stress switch so you can replenish and balance yourself before stress gets out of control?

What do you do to rejuvenate yourself and replenish your nutrient supplies (other than get your hair and nails done, getting a massage or eating a pint of ice cream)?

In this exercise, the focus is to simply increase your awareness of what is going on when your body/mind is relaxed and when you're stressed. You'll discover your key triggers and figure out how to control resistant stress, so you can regain balance more quickly and easily.

### Step 1

Take the next few days to simply start to bring more awareness to your body/mind when you are feeling relaxed. This may even be when you feel bored. Many of the women I work with are bored when they are not worrying or anxious about something so they find things to worry about or clean, just to stay busy. Maybe that's you, then again you know how to relax and what you need, you just need to do it more often. Make some metal notes or if you really want to get more accurate records, keep a journal on the extra space I left you here in this book.

Because the way we tend to remember things is not always the way it actually happened.

## Step 2

Now that you have something relaxing to weigh your stress levels against, start making notes of how your body/mind reacts to stress. Which of the Sources of Stress triggers your reactions most? How do you respond? What happens first, second, third? How long does it last? Then release tensions that tension & stress with what was relaxing in step 1, and if you can't apply it now, what have you done in the past that really helped you to let go and exhale your stress?

I'm hoping that if you've decided to purchase & read this book, you've also decided to actually take action to turn your stress around, instead of just reading along, believing that the solution to your stress will just seep into your brain via osmosis through reading alone. Trust me. I've tried that approach and it just doesn't work as well as you might hope. To create long lasting change, our peace of mind and personal self-worth need to be a priority. We actually need to play with these experiments on our own for at least 7-10 days consistently to discover what works.

So go ahead and play. Be your own living breathing experiment. You are free from right or wrong answers here… There are only observations.

**Have fun, take your time and experiment** with some solutions that have worked for you in the past that we may not have discussed her so far. You already know what works and **consistency is the key to success!**

**Use the space below to make some notes on your personal experimentation with stress.** This will allow you to make any necessary adjustments and have a clearer idea of how it affects you, as well as how to mindfully manage it...

# COACHING SESSION 6:
## *We Digest What?!*

So we left off discussing the definition of stress, the three stages of stress, as well as the sources of stress, and started to increase our awareness of how it affected, us as well as what to do about it.

Now I want to ask you a personal question...

How do you eat? You're probably thinking, "With my mouth". And yes, we all eat, but HOW we eat, can be a very personal and insightful thing to know. It can set the pace for our day, our energy levels, even our self-esteem and self-image. Would you consider yourself a fast eater or a slow eater? Maybe you are a distracted eater and focus on other things as you eat, such as the project you're involved in, or driving your car, or focused on Facebook. Then again, maybe you're the type of person who's typically standing, walking or rushing around while eating, doing your best to multi-task, literally shoving everything in at once, just to save time. Does any of this sound familiar?

When was the last time you ate a meal, and had a foodgasm? We've all had them at one time or another, no matter what our age. In fact, I've even seen toddlers experience a foodgasm when they discover a new food and are offered it again. A foodgasm is when your sense of pleasure becomes heightened the moment you simply think of having a specific food and your eyes connect with it as it is presented to you; your level of anticipation of having this food is greatly increased as you visually take in the details of it's color and its presentation. So much so, that your stomach aches for a taste. As you inhale the aroma of this masterpiece, it completely intoxicates you, making your mouth water; as its texture passes over your lips, and reaches your tongue, its taste lingers seductively in your mouth, bite after tantalizing bite, causing you inhale with sheer pleasure and let out a deep, meaningful sigh at the exquisiteness of it all. You pause and breathe for just a moment to let the moment last a bit longer, then continue on to the next round of seduction with the next bite. And this lasts until you've had enough, not because your plate is clean, but because it's just THAT satisfying you may only need a few bites.

(I'll give you a moment to really think about this, and catch your breath.)

Eating in this matter is relaxed and enjoyable, wouldn't you say? Imagine what it would be like if you ate at least one meal a day like this!

How often do you currently eat a meal in a casual, relaxed manor, where your senses, from the sight of your food to the smell and the taste, give you such satisfaction, you get to enjoy a little foodgasm with each and every bite? And yes, I know what you're thinking, "Who has time to eat like that?", or if you've actually never had that much enjoyment with your food, you might be thinking, "I'll have what she's having!"

I can assure you, that you do have time to get this much pleasure from your food. You can slow down, receive long lasting satisfaction and pleasure from the experience and still accomplish what's on your 'To Do' list, just as you did before when you were rushing around, maybe even better. Imagine how much more relaxed and reenergized you could be if you simply gave yourself 5 minutes to enjoy your food before rushing out the door. Time yourself, 5 minutes is longer than you may think.

We all seem to have it ingrained in our heads that WHAT we eat is important. And it is. What we eat can make a big difference in how we handle the triggers of our stress and various other events in our lives in a more proactive, productive way. Yet, HOW we eat plays a bigger role in our ability to receive the optimal nutrition from all those healthy foods we spend so much money on, in an effort to improve our health. How we eat effectively improves a wide variety of digestive challenges, general health imbalances, gives us longer lasting energy, plus it uplifts and stabilizes our moods. If we're paying attention, we may even find we're naturally eating less, while receiving more fulfillment, without having to put much effort into it at all; just increased our awareness.

Now let's talk specifically about the affects of our thoughts and stress on our digestion (which, by the way, is where up to 70% of our immune system is housed).

Let's begin by understanding digestion. There are actually a couple of definitions to this word, and I think that's just fabulous! Digestion is so much more than just the physical action we've been taught. The variety of its definitions give us a clue to its completeness. Those definitions are: "to obtain information, ideas, or principles"; "to assimilate mentally as well as to arrange methodically in the mind"; "to think over, such as when digesting an idea"; "to process a feeling into consciousness" and "the biological process that enables food to be converted into substances that can be absorbed and assimilated by the body".

How fascinating is that!? Digestion is so much a part of everything we think, feel and do every day! It's goes far beyond just the idea of taking in a carrot, chewing it, and breaking it down into nutrients the body can use as fuel, then discarding the waste. How we understand the world around us, every thought and feeling we have, as well as every decision we make, is taken in, broken down, processed, and compartmentalized in a matter of seconds to determine our feelings, reactions, and our actions to experiences around us. Sorting out the nurturing and nourishing from the toxic and lethal.

Kinda blows your mind doesn't it?

Here's something else; as we're eating, we digest every thought we're thinking, and emotion we're feeling, as well as the food we're consuming at the time. It's the synergy of our thoughts, feelings and food quality that influences whether we will be nourished or malnourished; energized through optimal digestion or lethargic and bloated due to indigestion. How many times a day do you sit down to eat while feeling a bit overwhelmed or stressed out? Before you even took a bite, were you adding up calories, points, grams of this, ounces of that or had some sort of negative thought about yourself playing in the background? Were your thoughts wrapped around something that happened in the past or anxious about something  in the future? Perhaps, it was a mental movie of an uncomfortable situation running through your mind as you sat down and started soothing yourself with your favorite comfort food. And after a little while, maybe you didn't feel so good anymore. Your stomach was in knots, maybe you were even feeling a bit bloated.

"Nature has provided us really with only two signals to be aware of: a sense of comfort and a sense of discomfort- and these can be physical, emotional or psychological" according to Deepak Chopra in his book, Perfect Digestion. How are you paying attention to these subtle messengers of digestive health?   What have you learned from them?

Every day we digest food, information, emotions, energy and so much more, yet we typically pay very little attention to it. Its only if we're uncomfortable, that it gets our attention, and even then, we tend to go about our day dealing with the discomfort by using an over the counter medicine to numb the pain, or we simply push through it attempting to ignore it. We hardly ever acknowledge when our digestion is in balance, because we typically take it for granted when we don't feel pain. Why is that? What could we learn by paying closer attention to the essential wisdom of our gut feelings, especially when they are in balance? Our gut intelligence is wise beyond the years of our educated minds. So why are we not paying closer attention to all it has to teach us?

Let me put it this way, have you ever felt a strong "gut feeling" about something? Ever had stomach cramps before a presentation? A "gut-wrenching experience"? What about butterflies in your stomach? Very few people ever say they had "a kidney feeling" or "a spleen feeling". We say we have a GUT feeling because part of us is keenly aware of the intelligence there, whether we are consciously aware of it or not. And these gut feelings are no longer considered a fanciful notion, but are now understood as a physiological fact that science has finally caught up with, and can confirm. We really do have two brains-one in our skull, and one in our gut.

Inside our digestive system is something truly amazing and vitally important...it's called the "enteric nervous system" and it is considered to be our "gut brain". The ENS is located within the tissue lining along the esophagus, stomach, small intestine and colon. It is a rich and intricate network of proteins and neurochemicals that sends messages between neurons, and support cells like those found in our skulls brain. And because of its intricate circuitry, it can act independently, learn, remember and produce feelings.

Our gut brain can also sense and control events in other parts of the body, including the brain. Demonstrating how the two brains are interconnected, with one having the ability to affect the other. What is totally interesting about all of this, is that it was discovered that that there is more communication from our gut-brain to the brain in our skull, than the other way around. This would mean that it would truly benefit us to start listening to our gut more often, and to start trusting our Inner Nutrition Guru.

Especially when it is in balance, so we have a better understanding of how to keep it that way.

Scientists discovered that we have around 100 million neurons in our gut brain, which is more than is held in our central nervous system, and our central nervous system plays a major role in how our body functions. This means that there is tremendous untapped potential to intelligent digestive health.

And what's more, the amazing mind/body connection integrates the use of our highly intelligent unconscious mind into this process. Our unconscious mind is what governs all bodily functions, creative thinking, problem solving and mental habits, such as writing your name, driving a car, walking, smoking, or eating...habits you don't have to consciously focus your attention on to do. When we sit down to eat with our educated conscious minds, we focus most of our attention on analyzing, criticizing and thinking logically. This is where we sit and start counting calories, and grams of this or ounces of that. Nourishment is not always about logic, and it's certainly not about analyzing or criticizing. It's about learning to listening to and trust our gut, to know for certain, what would sustain and nourish us for the long haul, which may sometimes be physical food, or it could simply be mental/emotional food. Either way, balanced digestion is the magic key to more energy, better total health, improved self-esteem and true peace of mind.

Regardless of whether we are consuming food in the physical sense, taking in mental food (food for thought) or ingesting emotional food (for example, guilt or praise) we go through the same process.

So what is the process of digestion and how do we balance it?

For our purposes here, we're going to focus on digestion of physical food for a moment, although the other elements (mental/emotional) do overlap. We can go more in-depth in the other areas at another time, possibly a new downloadable class or a book, but for now let's just focus on physical digestion.

## Basically, digestion works like this:

We take in food, break it down, absorb what we need and get rid of what is toxic to us.

Digestive Process:

Ingestive- when we take in food

Digestive- when we break it down

Absorption- when we take what we want into the blood stream

Elimination- getting rid of toxins & waste

When we sit down and add a generous helping of stress to this process, we introduce an element that clogs up the works.

In my many years of personal research and experimentation, I've come to the understanding that the physical digestion food starts first and foremost in the mind, long before it ever actually touches our lips.

We just discussed how our thoughts could create an environment that will result in toxicity, malnourishment and indigestion, or a calm environment where relaxation, nourishment, and optimal digestion allow us to thrive.

What's more, is that our thoughts and feelings have a huge impact on what we choose to eat, as well as when, where and how we eat it. I wouldn't ever tell you what to do, you know your body so much better than I do, but I would like to suggest that before you eating anything, just pause for a moment and check in with yourself. Simply focus on your breath, and ask your gut what would nourish me?

Maybe your mouth is a bit dry and you need to be hydrated. Go grab a glass of water and enjoy every satisfying drop. Sometimes when we are dehydrated, we begin to experience thoughts that are more anxious, lose focus and crave sweets. So before taking any other action first, go for a refreshing glass of water. After all, our brains are made of up to 80% water and our bodies around 70% water-so hydrate and enjoy the recharge.

Are you getting a slight rumbling in your tummy and whole food is really what would nourish your body/mind, or is your yearning for something else that would be much more nurturing and nutritive emotionally?

**Here's a quick relaxation routine my clients and I go through to help us feel more relaxed. Inhale and check in with yourself, are you finding your thoughts are all over the place and you need to get centered again?**

Exhale with a deep sigh, and create distance between you and your thoughts. Send them far off into the distance. With each exhalation they go farther and farther away, all details becoming unclear, white and fuzzy even, becoming smaller and smaller, until you can no longer see or feel them.

Inhale again, and just feel your bellybutton. Notice how rhythmically your breath goes in and out at a pace that is just right for you. Notice your toes. Wiggle them around, just feeling sensations in them and the ground they are on. Stay here for a few rounds of breaths, and when you are ready, imagine seeing yourself on the movie screen in your mind. Notice where you are, what you are wearing, the expression on your face, if you are talking with someone or by yourself, if you are standing or sitting. Allow one thought to play out in your mind the way you would like to imagine it and your role in its outcome. Allow in all the details you can, from vibrant colors to robust sounds and the most empowering feelings. Breathe in, and be aware of where in your body you feel the good feelings that you feel. Now notice how it is spinning, forwards, backwards, to the right, to the left, and just allow it to spin faster and faster until this positive, peaceful, empowering feeling is so intense you just don't know if you can take any more happiness. Then lock this feeling in, by imagining a zip lock bag sealing it up for you to get to where you wish anytime.

Now take a moment to be in the present moment again. Ask yourself *what is real and true.* Then take a nourishing, positive action.


Checking in with ourselves in this way only takes a moment or two after a bit of practice. By doing it consistently, we prevent ourselves from becoming ensnared in thoughts of the past or wrapped up in worries of the future. We come back to the here and now, to place where we have the most control over our actions and reactions. Hence, we become in control of our digestion simply because we are more calm and centered.

Yes, stressful thoughts will pop-up from time to time. It's human nature to worry about things and have concerns. Each one of us will sometimes feel less fabulous one day than the day before. And yet, our thoughts are our choice. What we choose to take in and digest is up to us. Are we going to allow in the thoughts and foods that are toxic, leaving us feeling miserable, or do we choose to accept, embrace and completely digest the thoughts and foods that lift us up, nourish and energize us? At the end of the day, our health, happiness and over all well-being is our choice to make.

Digestion is so much more than just taking in physical food. The process is basically the same, whether it's thoughts, emotions or food. We take something in, break it down (or filter it), absorb what we want, and discard what we don't need. I realize this way of understanding digestion is different from what we've been taught. Many of us still have the old one dimensional view of digestion stuck in our minds, even after I explained the multiple forms of digestion, that often happen all at the same time. So, I ask you to just consider this information as "food for thought" and give yourself the opportunity to digest it for a while. Play with the idea. What feels right to you and what do you discover in your own experiments?

## **Take a Mindful Moment:**

Take a moment to tune into yourself and the present moment before you begin to eat. This helps you get away from thoughts of the past or the future and gives you the opportunity to enjoy your meal in a more relaxed and mindful way.

- Begin by observing your surroundings. What sights do you see? What colors jump out at you? What colors are more hidden?

- How does your body feel? Take a moment to exhale your tension, and inhale some relaxation. This is a great time to Stop & Do 10…10 mindful breaths to relax and soothe your body/mind.

Once you feel more grounded, and more in the present moment, take a moment to really tune into your needs in this moment. What would nourish you right now and make you feel whole? Is it food or something else? If it is food, and you have a clear answer as to what it is you need, once you have your food, really look at it.

Notice the colors, are they vibrant or dull? Inhale, let in the aroma of your food. Does it make your mouth water? Feel the texture of it on your teeth & tongue. Be in this moment right now. Notice how good it tastes. Put your fork down and breathe in and out between bites. Savor each bite like a lover until the taste is no longer satisfying. When finished, simply pack up the rest for another time.

Practice relaxing & savoring your food like this over the next 7-10 days, and keep notes that you can refer back to over and over again.

What do you notice begins to happen as you eat?

How do your portion sizes change?

Where do your thoughts go as you eat?

# COACHING SESSION 7:
## Stop Eating Your Stress

So we just finished talking about digestion and how it's really so much more than just the physical digestion of food we've all been taught. That how we think about, interpret & relate to the world around us can also be considered part of digestion as well. Now let's talk about stress, eating & digestion…

How many times have you eaten somewhere and the appearance of where you were eating didn't make you feel relaxed? Like, say, at a fast food joint. If our eating environment is unappealing, we tend to begin our meal with a negative mindset, because this lacking environment will mildly stress us out. And as we now know, that will then affect how we digest our food, as well as how efficiently we will burn calories. If you are someone who wants to burn calories more efficiently, I suggest becoming more mindful of your environment as well as what your gut has to say. It can make eating so much more of the enjoyable experience it can be, instead of the chore that it tends to become when we diet.

I understand that we don't always have the opportunity to eat outdoors or in the setting of our dreams. However, we do have the choice of noticing what we <u>do</u> enjoy about our environment, as well as the option of finding a more pleasing location. Maybe a place that is quieter, and more soothing. It might require us to put on headphones and listen to music that soothes us and makes us happy inside or listen to the sounds of nature if we can't be there. Maybe we focus on enjoying spending time with the people we are sharing a meal with. It's all about choice.

How we choose to see our environment and what we choose to allow into our lives. The power is in your mind.

Next, notice the appearance of your food. Does it look so appetizing you can't wait to eat it? Does the smell make your mouth water?

When we think of, smell or see food that is appealing to us we begin to salivate and release salivary amylase. This digestive enzyme helps us digest our food even before it reaches our stomachs. Which is a fabulous reason to chew our food completely, instead of inhaling our food practically whole, because it can make less work for our stomach during the process of digestion. That can mean less indigestion.

The speed, or pace, we eat also plays a vital role in how we digest our food. If we eat too quickly, we tend to trigger anxiety in our gut, making the balanced digestion of all that healthy food we so diligently eat, practically null and void. In not so many words, the vital vitamins & nutrients in those foods get eliminated straight down the toilet.

We all have it ingrained into our heads that WHAT we eat is important. In contrast, HOW we eat plays a bigger role in our ability to digest, assimilate and metabolize our meal. HOW we eat can be a foodgasmic experience our whole body can benefit from!

HOW we eat affects all of our body systems, from our nervous system, to our digestion & elimination. They rely absolutely and completely on our central nervous system for optimal functioning.

Our central nervous system is like Grand Central Station for all other functions to travel through. Within our CNS (central nervous system), one specific section has the greatest influence on our digestion. This is called the Autonomic Nervous System.

Our ANS, can be broken down to into two subdivisions: our Sympathetic Nervous System and our Parasympathetic

Nervous System, which act as off-on switches for digestion. To make it a little easier, it may help to think of it like this: Each of our bodies are a unique corporation. Within that corporation, there is the main division that is in charge of all the inner workings and over sees operations (our CNS), constantly doing its best to maintain balance within. The Central Nervous System can't do everything well so rather than getting overloaded; they created a specialized division that is in charge of only digestion (our ANS or autonomic nervous system). That division is so specialized, it too didn't want to become overloaded with any extra work, so it divided itself into two specialized sub-sections. One that turns digestion off when there is a threat, otherwise known as stress (sympathetic nervous system), and one to turn it back on when that threat is gone (parasympathetic nervous system). Together they all work in harmony, like a well-oiled machine, constantly striving for homeostasis, otherwise known as balance... unless we come along with our mindless, rushed, stressed out eating and clog up the works.

## Here's what happens when we eat with stress:

- Digestion is turned off

- Decrease of oxygen to the belly, which robs our bodies of vital nutrients

- Nutrients that we do receive are not getting where they need to be, due to less enzymatic production

- We eliminate nutrients through our urine...calcium, magnesium, chromium, zinc, selenium...

- Messages are sent to the body to store food as fat and stop building muscle

When we eat due to stress, or with stress as our companion, our digestion gets turned off. After all, who would want to take the time to eat cookies, ice cream, chips or anything else if they feel threatened? Digestion isn't really necessary in a fight or flight situation. Our energy would really serve us better in other places, don't you think? Yet, majorities of women in America today all seem to eat with stress as their constant companion by running out the door, feeling the pressure of the clock at their heels with food hanging out of our mouths. Eating & drinking a full meal as we drive the car, to at least be able to say that we ate, and my personal favorite. eating while standing and taking care of everyone else's needs.

---

**Digestion Is OFF-** When your Sympathetic Nervous System is Dominant. Your body/mind is stressed (fight flight, or freeze) and digestion is suppressed.

**Digestion Is ON-** When your Parasympathetic Nervous System is Dominant. Your body/mind is relaxed and digestion is activated & more powerful.

---

This natural stress response causes a decrease of oxygen to the belly, which robs our bodies of vital nutrients. The few nutrients we may receive don't get where they need to be, due to a decrease in enzymatic production. Consequently, we end up eliminating nutrients through our urine. We lose nutrients such as calcium, magnesium, chromium, zinc, selenium. Probably the same nutrients we may be taking already as a supplement to better manage our stress. Wouldn't it be nice to save some money by simply slowing down & eating nutrient dense foods?

Messages from the brain are sent to the body to store food as fat and stop building muscle. Ugh! No wonder we have muffin tops! We're storing our fat for a day we feel less stressed! We think when will that day come and how long will it last? I don't know, you may be thinking. Well, when do you want it to be here? How would you know when you were relaxed? When we're stressed, we also tend to skip meals. Do you? Have you ever skipped a meal or meals when you were feeling pressured to get things done? How many times have you been so busy or preoccupied with something during the day that you don't eat because you feel as if there is no time, or because you just forgot?

Then later in the day, when things may be a bit less intense, our cravings start to kick in at full steam! Maybe we stop at a fast food place, wolf down some convenient foods such as crackers, chips, breads, pastas, a candy bar or an energy bar. Maybe it works for a little while, but then find that we're craving something else-not sure what- and we eat everything we can get our hands on, in an attempt to feel satiated. We reach for the very foods that can create emotional comfort for us and have a tumultuous love affair with them.

Studies have proven that this approach (of skipping meals, then binging on convenience foods later) creates more mood swings, depression and aggressive behavior than in those who eat regular meals made up of whole foods. In fact, the very comfort foods that raise our serotonin levels, and make us feel as if all is good with the world again, also tend to create more cravings, obesity, over eating, mental self-bashing and a whole host of physical health challenges ranging from digestive complaints to chronic joint pain and more.

Convenience foods are just that, convenient. They are also incomplete and create cravings. You see, as we eat these refined foods, they create a spike in our blood sugar levels and we get an instant rush of pleasure, as well as glucose.

After a few minutes, that rush wears off and we're left with deeper feelings of anxiety, despair and loss than we felt before eating those comfort foods in the first place. This happens because a sudden rush of insulin needs to be released into the blood, in the same way water from a fire hose rushes to put out a fire, just to help stabilize the amount of sugar now in our system. To top it all off, those sweet treats many of us love, rob our bodies of the very nutrients that would satisfy our cravings for nourishment to feel better longer, and help us better manage our stress in the first place and its higher nutrient dense foods that are our friends when it comes to reducing stress & stress eating. Therefore, the trick is to simply start crowding out some of our old hurtful acquaintances, and start introducing ourselves to some new best friends.

Our American lifestyle consists of so few whole foods created by Mother Nature, that in order for us to reduce the effects of this lifestyle such as diabetes, obesity and raised blood pressure- the weight loss industry has created a convenient way to help people on diets with the very same convenient, incomplete foods, thus creating more cravings in the process and more money in their bank accounts.

## So what's the solution?

When do we stop abusing ourselves and start nourishing ourselves instead? What is it going to take to start listening to our unique needs with greater awareness, then follow through, and give ourselves what we REALLY need?

Before we can effectively stop eating our stress, we need to learn what our stress triggers are and how to better manage our stress. This will create a more nourishing relationship between you and yourself as well as the foundation to creating a life that is simpler, more enjoyable and totally in your control.

When I was learning how to put the puzzle pieces together and transform my personal stress years ago, I started by making a conscious decision to never let stress get the better of me again. I was tired of feeling like a victim in my life, and being prisoner to my anxieties. Maybe you're making the same promise to yourself now. When I first started, it took a lot of trial and error to figure out what was the perfect fit for my unique needs and me at that time. You know what, because we are organic, natural beings, we are constantly changing and evolving. Therefore, our unique needs are changing and evolving as well. The journey towards this discovery can be fascinating instead of a struggle. Here's an opportunity to give ourselves the attention we may be craving and learn so much about ourselves.

I would be lying to you if I told you this was effortless. I would be lying if I told you change would happen over night. The truth is, genuine transformation is not fast, effortless or easy. However, it is simple. We get out of life whatever we put into it and the same holds true for our self-care. We tend to spend so much energy focusing our time, attention and love on others and leave ourselves depleted, craving the same attention and care in return. So what's really stopping us from giving ourselves what we're seeking? Imagine what would your life look like if you felt more confident & comfortable with yourself and truly loved whom you were inside and out. How would it feel to know you could actually do and be whatever you wanted, simply because you believed you could? I believe one of the reasons stress, anxiety and depression have the ability to mentally imprison us, is because on some level, we stopped believing in ourselves. How could a stressful or depressed moment shift for you, if instead of asking yourself, "Why me?" you checked in with your priorities and asked "What would truly nourish me in my heart & soul?". How could things be different if you took a few calming breaths before lashing out at your kids for not listening to you? How much nicer could your drive to work be, if instead of spending your time replaying stressful thoughts about your day over and over, you offered yourself a different perspective? One that included what was possible and made you feel good, instead of what sucks and isn't going so well? What would happen if instead of rushing out the door in the morning with a cup of coffee and a piece of toast, you made the time to enjoy a small breakfast before you walked out the door? How could that influence your mood, your cravings later on in the day, your mindset?

I believe Positive Self T.A.L.K (Trust, Awareness/ Acceptance, Listening with Love, Kindness or Compassion) is the foundation to simplifying our lives, preventing our stress from taking over and uplifting our moods. It's been like a magic wand for so many of the women I work with. Repeatedly, it's proven to improve their relationships, their enjoyment at work, lowered their anxiety levels, changed eating habits and even prevented over eating. All because they chose to give themselves the attention, love and energy towards self-care they deserved, instead of allowing the criticizing, abusive voice within to wear them down with "should", "have to", "try" and so on.

We can prevent stress & anxiety from capturing us. We have the power to end our mindless, reactive form of eating and over eating. It just takes a bit of mindfulness and self-love. By eating in a relaxed, comfortable & mindful way, we turn on powerful digestion, experience more pleasure during our meal, receive the essential nutrients we need to thrive and prevent over eating.

## HOW ARE YOU EATING?

I said it before, and I'll say it again...most Americans are not starving by any means. Except, they are malnourished due to the low quality of foods they are choosing and the stressful way in which they are eating. By eating our food in a pleasing environment and in a relaxed, pleasurable way, not only do we improve our digestion, the assimilation of nutrients and the elimination of toxins, it brings more vitality and joy to our lives! Food is a social element to any occasion, family meals, dates, parties, weddings, holidays and so on. It's part of family traditions, a connection to those who love us and so much more. So it's no wonder so many of us crave the very foods at bring us comfort when we are stressed, depressed or lonely.

## Take a Mindful Moment:

**Step 1**-Take a moment now to simply observe and bring greater awareness to your body/mind to find out if stress is your companion.

Where are you tense and tight?

Is your jaw clenched?

Shoulders tight and up around your ears?

How is your breathing?

Are you breathing from your chest or from your belly?

This simple awareness can help reduce stress levels immediately. Once we bring our awareness into the now, we can do something about it. Our thoughts when we are stress, anxious or worried are usually tangled up in thoughts of the past or the future. Things that have happened we berate ourselves for or obsess over what someone else did, or we are worried about what will come.

When we bring our awareness into this moment right now, how we are feeling, how we are breathing, hearing the breath going in and out of our bodies. Seeing the color and the sights around us, we get ourselves out of this trance like state of anxiety, stress and worry back into the present moment. Play with this for a few days before you go on to the next step.

*What do you discover?*

**Step 2**-Bring the same awareness you practiced earlier to the table with you now. As you sit down to your meal, where are your thoughts focused? Are you tangled up in the past, somewhere off into the future or are you in the present moment right now, aware of the scenery around you, the sounds and the smells?

Check in with yourself. How does your body feel? Where are you tight & tense? Where are you breathing from? Your chest or your belly? Focusing on exhaling first, and letting go of what you don't need helps us inhale and receive greater relaxation more easily. Exhale between 5-10 breaths. Notice the subtle shift of relaxation in your body. Notice there is a bit more clarity to your thinking as you come into the present.

What would truly nourish you right now? Listen to your inner nutrition wisdom. Before you order your food, or make your selection, imagine what it would taste like if you ate it. How does it satisfy your taste buds? Now imagine how it feels 15 minutes to an hour later AFTER eating that food. How do you feel about your choice? How does your body feel? Are you vibrant & energized or tired and moody?

Play with this for a few days then go onto the next step. Establishing great awareness of your needs and the effects of your choices in this way will have a great pay off in the long run. You are establishing a trusting, loving and compassionate relationship with yourself through simple awareness, something that may be missing in your life.

# SOME MORE MINDFUL
# STRESS SOLUTIONS

## Solution 1- Reframe Your Stress!

Stress. It can feel so overwhelming it brings you to your knees, and gets you bawling in the bathroom until all the tissues and toilet paper are gone. Then when the crying is over, and we are feel completely drained, we take in a few cleansing breaths and let go of all the crap until we have our composure back. This my friend is the perfect opportunity to change how we perceive the event in our mind. Create more clarity and set into motion a truer, healthier and more empowering course of action. Our minds are amazing and I am constantly in awe of how powerful they are. After all our reality, our world and everything in it is contrived in our minds. Life is exactly how we perceive it to be, and we have the power to alter that perception with a few quick steps.

There have been many times in my life when someone said something, maybe a boss, a friend or a family member that really just cut to the quick. Completely tore me up inside. I really had to check in with myself to figure out if my perception of the situation was accurate or if I was interpreting it in a way that was definitely not beneficial for me. That's usually the time I make a few adjustments in my thinking to get a better perspective so I can carry on with my day, in my typical happy, easygoing way.

Here's what I do...ready? You may think it's overly simplified, but when you do it yourself, you may discover how powerfully it works. Simple is really the best way to go. Ok, for real this time...Here's what I do...I pay attention to, and step away from, the voice I'm hearing speak to me in my mind over & over as I recall the conversation. The one that is being critical, bashing me or stressing me out. Then I create the image of the person the voice is connected to, making sure I get all the details.

Next, I imagine that I'm holding a magic remote control. With this magic remote, I change the sound of their voice. Making them sound funny, as if they just sucked in an entire balloon full of helium, and they now sound just like Minnie Mouse. I'll also use my remote control to adjust their outfit so they're now wearing oversized clown clothes and a clown nose as they are talking to me, and sometimes I'll add in a mohawk with bright rainbow colors for good measure. Then I will attempt to play back the event in my mind and not laugh. I'll even imagine the event being played in rewind with all the high-pitched sounds and crazy outfits. When I'm done with my fun, I imagine that the TV in my mind is being turned off and the picture drains of all its color and shrinks down to a speck then disappears.

By the time I'm done with my moment I have a clearer perspective and a better understanding of the situation. Many times, I am simply better able to just let it go. Because what I realize, is that the other person's reaction may not be due directly to what I did or said, but to how they are interpreting the world themselves. Sometimes they need a little perspective as well.

## Solution 2- Stop & Do 10!

In a world that seems to always be asking you to give more and more of yourself every day, we need time to give back to ourselves. We need time to recharge and it can take all of 10 full seconds to do it. If you want to completely indulge yourself, you could even make it an entire minute.

 Our breath is incredibly powerful and our entire existence depends on it. When we're stressed out, we tend to hold our breath or breathe so shallowly that it's as if we aren't breathing at all anyway. Creating all sorts of "symptoms", we may think we need medical attention when all we really need to do is take deep relaxing breaths into our belly button's.

I know a thing or two about this since I used to do exactly that, breathe so shallowly that I eventually would pass out and couldn't figure out why. Then after a bit of personal awareness, I realized that when I got stressed I would hold my breath for long periods or breathe incredibly shallow as if I was sipping air through a straw with one nostril. To remedy that and prevent my panic attacks I would do something very simple, and I often suggest to the women that I work with to do the same...STOP & DO 10.

## HERE'S HOW:

The moment you feel stressed, in your mind say "STOP!". Just stop when you're doing & thinking, and simply freeze. Bring your awareness inside. Now EXHALE out all the tension you're holding onto. Dump those garbage bags. Imagine what it would feel like to just let them go...INHALE and receive clean, fresh restorative oxygen. Imagine what it would feel like to receive complete peace and relaxation, as if you were on a tropical island vacation. Now begin counting on each exhalation- EXHALE (1) and let go of the toxic sludge you're holding onto. INHALE and receive peace. EXHALE (2) and free yourself from the vines holding you down...INHALE and be. EXHALE (3), imagine space opening up within you...INHALE, and receive vitality.

*Get the idea?*

Now it's Your Turn:

What is it going to take for you to STOP & DO 10 to turn your stress around? Doing this especially before eating activates powerful digestion and can reduce portion sizes, as well as help you receive the nutrients from your food for repair & maintenance of your nervous system

## Solution 3- Yoga, You & The Stress Monster

Yoga means to join together, union. With that in mind we understand that there is no separation between what we think, say, eat or do. They are all connected and so are each and every one of us. We are connected with each and every being, as well as every aspect of nature, from plants to bugs, the grass, the tress, the mountains and clouds. We are a microcosm of the macrocosm. Yoga is wonderful at helping us create a more balanced and positive relationship with ourselves, as well as a more balanced, positive relationship with our food and the people around us. Each asana, or pose, strengthens the body and the mind. It brings us to our core, to our center and aligns us with our highest intentions. Introducing more calm, balance and well-being into our lives gently and easily, which overflows to the people we know and care for. Eventually we are able to Be The Change We Wish To See In The World, as Ghandi suggested. All because we allowed that change to start from within, with an awareness of what makes you unique within this intricate web of life, and how your thoughts and actions affect the world around you. There are varieties of forms of yoga to practice to fit each and every person. Some yoga styles are gentle and move slowly, allowing the practitioner to experience each and every pose such as in Hatha yoga. Another style known as Vinyasa, or "flow yoga", is fast paced and intense. There is lively music that plays and will definitely let you test your physical limits if that is what you are looking for. A Restorative class is what I typically suggest to my clients because it is a delicious introduction to yoga and so easy to do. It incorporates bolsters, blankets and a variety of other props so the student can passively relax into each and every pose for deep restoration on a cellular level. In fact, a good restorative class is more beneficial than any nap. I've barely touched the surface of what styles of yoga are available, and if you are interested, visit The Yoga Journal online for more information. From personal experience, I can assure you that yoga can play a large role in how you manage your stress. Every client who I refer to a restorative class comes back grateful they attended. If you are shy about going to a class Rodney Yee has some wonderful videos you can purchase and do at home. He is great for the person who is new to yoga and curious. I also love the full classes you can take part in from Kripalu. Just visit kripalu.org or visit vimeo.com and search for "Kripalu yoga" to discover for yourself how relaxing and restorative it can be! However, I do suggest that you take a few classes at your local yoga studio, so your teacher can help you with proper alignment. It would be rather stressful to get hurt doing something that was meant to relax, restore and rejuvenate you. Personally I prefer the videos as a way to include yoga into my day according to my schedule, when I just am not able to make it to a live class.

Recently, I had been at one of the yoga studios I work from, and had been talking with Ellen Mackay, an experienced yoga teacher, who teaches a variety of yoga classes from Vinyasa to Restorative, about suggestions for relieving stress during the day. She suggested two simple things to do that help you unwind, chill out and rest more easily both during the day and at night. **A Shoulder Shrug** and **Supported Savasana.**

For the **Shoulder Shrug**, she suggests that you sit comfortably in a chair or on your yoga mat. Rest your hands, palms up, on your thighs. As you inhale, draw your shoulders up towards your ears. As you exhale through your mouth making a "Ha" sound, let the shoulders drop down. Repeat with each breath and begin to notice the shoulders, neck and jaw begin to relax. She recommends following your breath for at least five exhalations to receive all the benefits from this exercise. It can be done anywhere from your car, the train the checkout line to your desk, and obviously at home. Give it a go right now, what differences in your stress and tension do you notice? Any shifts in your mental focus?

For **Supported Savasana**, she suggests that for at least 3 minutes you lie down on your bed or yoga mat, bringing a bolster or two pillows under your knees. She suggests you can also use a pillow under your head, if your neck needs more support. Once in position, let your arms rest out to the sides, with your palms up. Allow the muscles in your face to relax and maybe begin to close the eyes. If your eyes do not close naturally, you can use an eye pillow or a folded towel over the eyes to help relax the face muscles.

Begin to notice your breath moving in and out through your nose. Imagine as if that breath is a healing light and allow the light to move to all the muscles in the body, bringing in relaxation and releasing tension. I have done this many times at bedtime after having a bit of chamomile tea and find myself resting deeply and soundly during the night.

When I moved to Florida a few years ago with my family, Ellen's classes were the first I took. She has a great knowledge of yoga and is a fantastic teacher who truly cares about her students, and because of this she has quite the local following. If you live in the Riverview Florida area, I suggest checking out one of her classes. I promise you'll be glad you did!

There are two more poses you can easily do at home, that require no major instruction, **Child's Pose** and **Downward Dog**. I find myself doing these periodically throughout my day, when I feel a little tense or just need a break. They both offer an emotional haven to let go of what I've tangled myself up in to simply be & breathe. To get into **Child's Pose**, get onto all fours on the floor and sit back on your heels (if your behind doesn't reach your heels you can put a blanket there to help). Bend towards the floor, resting your forehead onto the floor with your arms resting along the side of you or stretched in front of you. You can also rest your forehead on crossed arms in front of you if that is more comfortable. Then simply let go and breathe into your belly. This pose allows us to feel safe and protected as if we are back in our mother's womb. It helps loosen muscles in the lower torso that can get tight and stimulates our Sacral Chakra (2nd).

For **Downward Dog** you'll again get onto all fours on the floor, spreading the fingers to create a stable base. Tuck your toes under, so the balls of your feet now have a little weight on them, push your hips up, and lift your knees off the floor. In this pose, you now look like a tee-pee. Relax your neck and head, maybe gently swinging them side to side or front to back to help loosen them up. Send your chest towards your legs as far as they will comfortably go, stretching the spine as you lengthen and extend the arms, guiding the tailbone backward and upward. Breathe into your belly, and exhale fully and completely with a deep sigh. This pose enables us to relax, stretch and feel the joy and playfulness of our own bodies. It energizes the Heart Chakra (4th) and help us release and let go of to unwanted attachments.

When I am feeling tense, overwhelmed and as if I am giving to everyone except myself, it is not uncommon to see me stop what I am doing and go through a few yoga poses. A favorite of mine, that helps to open up the Solar Plexus Chakra, (whose imbalance is often connected digestive complaints, stress and low self-esteem) is the **Lion's Roar**. It's wonderful for releasing stress, fear, frustration & irritation. Mainly because it is **a powerful breathing technique that helps let us let go of all the tension and emotions we tend to store in our jaw, throat & belly without realizing it.** Here's how you do it: Find a quiet spot where you can be alone for about 5 minutes. Then sit on your heels with your back straight.

Next, put your hands on the floor in front of you, with your fingers pointing backwards. Inhale deeply into your belly allowing it to fully expand. Simply observe the sensations you feel as you connect with your breath, then let open your mouth and let your tongue hang out as you exhale completely and roar like a lion, releasing all those pent up emotions and tensions in your belly, throat and jaw. Sit for a moment to observer the change in your body then repeat  again this several times. Breathing into your belly, connecting with your breath and powerfully releasing any unwanted stress, tension & emotions. Stop when you feel drained of what you no longer need. Enjoy the lightness and power that begins to circulate.

## Are yoga poses not your thing yet?

Ayurveda, the traditional medicinal healing system of India, suggests that to unwind and let go of stress, dim the lights in the house as the sun begins to set. This signals the body/mind that the frenetic pace you've been going at all day can came to an end. That's it's time to "turn off". This includes all electronic devices as well. By turning off all electronics an hour or two before bed and winding down with a book or quality family time we uplift our spirits and naturally recharge. You may even want to include soothing, aromatic scents of sandalwood or vanilla incense (or a few drops of aromatherapy oils to a bath or room diffuser). These aromas are grounding, balancing and calming. When we consistently use these scents during a time of relaxation, we create an association with them, so whenever we smell that certain aroma, we automatically know to relax. This means we can use these scents when we need them, wherever we go…and this includes traveling.

Here's a small note about essential oils. Not all oils are created the same. The industry is not highly regulated and the oils we can buy at our favorite health food store for very little money, tend to be mostly perfume oils. To receive the greatest benefits of these little gems, we need the highest quality oils because they organically infuse themselves into our bodies. If we are going to take the time to love & care for ourselves, to reduce our stress and emotional eating, and basically start making ourselves more of a priority, then ingestible, therapeutic grade oils are the way to go. So who can you count on? If you are going to choose a company, I highly recommend either DoTerra or Young Living Oils, because after years of personal research and experimentation, hands down there is no company like them. They are both high quality oils, ethically created and free of synthetic compounds or contaminates.

*Now back to Ayurveda recommendations....*

Ayurveda also suggests a warm beverage at the end of the day, maybe even during that relaxing hour right before bed. Traditionally it is recommended to heat a cup of organic, whole milk until it comes to a gentle rolling boil. Add in a pinch of nutmeg, cardamom (both said to promote sleep) along with cinnamon (for digestion) and honey to taste. If you don't drink milk then sipping chamomile, lemon balm or Valerian tea can offer the same soothing feeling.

Finally, I'm going to talk about the breath again, this time from an Ayurvedic perspective. Two of the best ways to center yourself during the day, when you need a moment to yourself, is with the **Three-Part Breath** (Dirga Pranayama) **Alternate Nostril Breathing** (Pranayama). These practices help to calm the nervous system and center the mind. To begin the **Three-Part Breath**, simply sit comfortably in a chair, with your spine straight, yet relaxed. Place your hands in your lap face up or face down, whichever is most comfortable to you. Inhale and exhale a few breaths, in and out through your nose, just focusing on the sound and feel of your breath. Notice your shoulders, your jaw and muscles in your face. As you feel ready, begin to deepen your breath into your belly, being sure to only breathe into the belly with relaxed shoulders. You are free from any straining or struggling for breath. Now, relax your jaw, noticing the space between the back teeth and your tongue. As you continue to breathe in and out through your nose, notice how your breath begins to easily move through your belly, ribs and chest. Notice how relaxed your shoulders, your throat, your jaw and face muscles are... and if the mind wanders, simply bring your focus back to your inhale and exhale into your belly, then your ribs and finally your chest both front and back. You will be breathing fully and completely in a relaxed, rhythmic way that is best for you.

To practice **Pranayama**, simply hold out your hand and close your index and middle finger into your hand. Place your right thumb over your right nostril closing off the airway. Inhale through your left nostril, then using your ring finger, close off the left nostril as you lift off your thumb and inhale through your right nostril, alternating between sides flowing from right to left and left to right. Do this all the while breathing into your nostril down into your belly. 5-10 rounds are all it takes and is a great way to transition from hectic activity to peaceful stillness.

### Now It's Your Turn:

Where will you get started? Will you start with alternate nostril breathing and some aromatic scents or will you dim the lights and turn off all electronics after getting into child's pose or supported Savasana?

Here's your opportunity to play with, and discover what nourishes you for total and natural relaxation.

## Solution 4- Let's Get Physical!

Sex. Now that's something physical isn't it? It gets your body moving, your blood pumping, raise serotonin & dopamine levels and can give you a great work out. However, it's not always convenient or acceptable to do in public. Therefore, there are other options that can be just as fun.

That is really the point of being physically active, isn't it? To have fun that makes us feel like a kid again! So many times we take part in activities that we really have little or no interest in, all in the name of exercise and getting fit. That is very commendable, but stressful. If we need to drag ourselves out the door every time to get to the gym or wherever we go for exercise, then we are triggering our stress response, and part of the whole point of exercising is to release happy endorphins and let go of stress. So what are some things you liked to play as a kid? Do you like to dance? How about swimming? Maybe you can come up with a whole bunch of reasons why you can't do those things-that's fine. It's your mindset, and your life. How has that thinking helped you so far?

And we both know, that where there is a will, there is a way. Dance around your house to music you love, engage your kids, your husband, your pet and dance with them! Join your local YMCA and go swimming. Walk around the block every night after dinner and make it a family affair or invite your neighbors. Be creative and playful, just like you were as a child. There are so many ways to get your body moving and work off that stress! A client of mine put a punching bag in her office. She has little sparring matches with the punching bag before she goes to lunch, to work off her tension, instead of bringing it to the table with her. I love playing freeze tag and going on adventure walks with my daughter. We make the adventure walk like a scavenger hunt and often walk miles without realizing it, simply because we had so much fun. I also enjoy swimming, hiking, kayaking and especially yoga. By the end of whatever I'm doing, I'm completely relaxed, refocused and totally rejuvenated. However, if you enjoy going to the gym, go! If you like taking classes, and find yourself only working out on the machines, find classes that interest you. I understand Zumba is a lot of fun, and really gives you a great workout!

### How will you get moving?

When and where can you see yourself fitting it into your life?

What benefits do you notice in your mindset after you've really had a great workout?

How does your reaction to stressful situations change?

What shifts in your eating habits occur for the better?

How do you feel about yourself after a week, a month or six of activity?

## Solution 5- Foods & Mood, prevent imbalance, instead of fighting it.

As I've mentioned before food does play a role in our moods and in how we manage or prevent our stress. Many things such as our blood sugar levels, neuro-nutrients (which are vitamins & minerals that impact brain function) and our breath affect our moods. It can take years of nutrient depraved eating habits before the consequences of those habits emerge, and by that time, they could be pretty severe. I found this out first hand. After years of living on very few whole foods, lots of caffeine, sugar, alcohol and processed foods when I was younger, I eventually had consistent, "grand-mal seizure" looking convulsions that no one could figure out the cause of. I'd been to specialists who had given me every test they could come up with at the time, yet they couldn't figure out the cause and eventually told me it was all in my head. They then prescribed me some medication to control them. It wasn't until I decided to take responsibility for the results of my actions that I realized my eating habits, as well as how I was thinking, all contributed to those "seizures" manifesting. In the end, I became my own living experiment, which is how I came upon many of the experiments I had you go through as you read the book. They were actually some of the steps I took to find balance physically, mentally & emotionally in my own life.

When we are nutrient deprived, the first signs of imbalance are a shift in mood. Which to be honest can be slight, so we rarely pay attention to them, and tend to head to the coffee machine or the snack machine if we unconsciously notice it. According to the author of The Food-Mood Solution, Jack Challem being mindful of our changes in mood and behavior can be the key to understanding the strong association with a person's physical health. He goes on to give this example-"people who are depressed are more likely than non-depressed individuals to develop heart disease or cancer, and quick-tempered men are more likely than others to drop dead from sudden heart attacks."

Our mind & body are intricately connected. What goes on in the mind will be seen in the body and what goes on in the body will be reflected in the mind. When we are nutrient deprived, we set off a domino effect of imbalances because the same blood that flows through the body also flows through the brain that Carrying nutrients that either uplift, empower and energize us or do just the opposite.

So after going through my own research, I've included some of the foods you can eat that can help you prevent malnutrition in both body & mind and reduce the effects of stress-because as we now know, malnutrition doesn't just happen in third world countries, it happens here at home too.

According to Dr Andrew Saul from the film Food Matters, two handfuls of **raw cashews** provides the equivalent mood boosting effects as a therapeutic dose of Prozac. Isn't that awesome? Raw cashews are one of the highest natural sources of tryptophan, which is the precursor for the production of serotonin (the feel good hormone) in the brain.

While I'm talking about nuts, let's consider the **Almond**. They have been over looked for far too long as a stress relieving food. Almonds contain zinc, as well as iron. Zinc is a key nutrient for maintaining a balanced mood, and iron can prevent brain fatigue, which has been found to contribute to both anxiety and a lack of energy.

Researchers have found **blueberries** to be rich in vitamins, a variety of antioxidants as well as phytonutrients, that are considered extremely beneficial for relieving stress.

**Peaches** contain a natural sedative that helps to reduce stress and anxiety and can actually help to induce sleep if eaten before we go to bed.

**Dark Chocolate** is awesome. I don't think I've ever met someone who doesn't like chocolate. Even Dr. Mercola endorses it (click here to read his article). Dark chocolate contain the amino acid Tryptophan, which as I mentioned earlier with the cashews, is the precursor for the production of serotonin (the feel good hormone) in the brain. It also contains Theobromine, which is the ingredient that is toxic to dogs, but recent studies have shown that has a positive, mood elevating effect on those that ingest it. It also has Magnesium, and if you are a supplement taker, with stress you are probably taking a magnesium supplement to manage your stress. Magnesium helps to relieve anxiety, nervousness, spasm and tics. Although it's best to take magnesium with calcium, avoid milk chocolate. It's really only chocolate flavored sugar and isn't very helpful at all when looking to replace lost nutrients during stress and anxiety.

**Leafy Greens**. Really, I've nothing left to say except eat your greens. Leafy greens are the least consumed food in America. Which is really SAD, because leafy greens are **so uplifting and contain everything we need to prevent and reduce anxiety, stress, depression as well as many of our health challenges**. In wholistic medicine, which is followed by many Asian cultures, they believe the color green is related to the liver, emotions and stability, as well as associated with springtime, vitality and renewal. "Greens help build our internal rainforest", as my teacher at the Institute for Integrative Nutrition Joshua Rosenthal said during class one day. And after making a conscious choice to add more greens into my daily menu, I can attest to that...and so can my clients. **So what's in these powerhouses?** Let me tell you. Leafy greens are naturally rich in calcium, magnesium, iron, potassium, phosphorous, zinc, vitamins A.C, E and  K and are crammed with fiber, folic acid, chlorophyll and a variety of  phytochemicals, antioxidants and many other micronutrients. Eat them raw, steamed, sautéed or in soups. However, you can introduce more of them into your menu the better you will feel!

## Natural Sweets for the Stressed Out.

We all crave sweets, but as I mentioned earlier, the quality of what we consume really matters. Therefore, I'm offering a few alternatives that will be sweet without robbing your body of essential nutrients.

**Date Sugar.** Made from dehydrated dates and finely ground keeping the fruits vitamins, minerals & fiber content, it's a good source of  minerals like calcium, iron, magnesium, phosphorus, zinc, copper, manganese, and selenium, which are essential to maintaining balance in body and mind.  It can be used directly on foods when baking, just keep in mind that it doesn't dissolve (I use it in my chocolate chip recipe instead of  white or brown sugar).

**Maple Syrup** is simply boiled down tree sap and an excellent source of manganese and a good source of zinc. It can be used as table sweetener on waffles, pancakes, or in baking to make cakes, breads, muffins, cookies, etc. Not recommended for regular use, as it can spike glucose levels, but it's rich in manganese & zinc and also contains calcium, potassium and copper, which are essential to maintain the normal metabolic activities in the body, so it's a better choice than table sugar.

**Organic Local Raw Honey** has anti-bacterial, anti-viral and anti-fungal properties. It is also being studied for its anti-cancer and anti-tumor properties. Heating destroys the substances responsible for these properties. Fresh, raw honey available in summer months, has friendly Lactobacilli (good intestinal bacteria), not found in winter months. Honey contains antioxidants that scavenge the free radicals from the body we create when stressed, reduces LDL (bad cholesterol) levels, relieves congestion in the upper respiratory tract and when taken along with ginger, also, improves digestion...BONUS!

**Brown Rice Syrup** tastes like butterscotch and has a low glycemic value, which means it does not cause a sugar rush or a sudden spike in blood sugar so it's also a better choice for people who need to watch their blood sugar levels. It's a good source of magnesium that helps in relieving fatigue, relaxing the muscles & nerves. Good source of potassium. Good source of iron. Additionally, it's a very good source of manganese and B-vitamins. These are all essential for a balanced mood. Tip: great to dip apples in instead of caramel!

**Stevia** does not affect blood sugar levels, so it's great for diabetics and people with glucose sensitivities; it's a natural anti-oxidant and rich in fiber. It contains most of the essential minerals and vitamins required for good health.

**A HUG.** A Hug has no calories at all, won't harmfully affect your glucose and can do so much more for you than just say hello or good-bye! A brief hug and 10 minutes of handholding with a romantic partner greatly reduce the harmful physical effects of stress, according to a study reported by the American Psychosomatic Society. Reaching out and touching someone, and holding them tight—is a way of saying you care. Its effects are immediate: for both, the hugger and the person being hugged, feel good.

According to Parveen Chopra, a pioneer in New Age journalism in India, and founder of the country's first body-mind-spirit monthly magazine *Life Positive*, Hugs are being used even as an aid in treating some physical illnesses, following research that discovered it leads to positive physiological changes. Because hugs affect our biochemistry. They raise our Endorphin levels (The body's natural painkiller); our Serotonin and Melatonin levels (The 'Happy Hormones') help make us feel loved, which makes everyone feel good! We have such an emotional connection to our foods especially to our sweets. When life is not sweet enough for us, when we have had too much stress or simply need reassurance-we tend to crave sweets... By taking the action to nourish & nurture yourself with a hug you are not only giving your emotions what you need, clearly you're a benefiting your chemistry as well. As I said before, this is a short list and I know you will be able to research for yourself and find many other foods that help you in preventing and managing your stress.

So Take A Mindful Moment!

Be your own experiment. Introduce more greens into you daily menu. Have two handfuls of raw cashews a day. Give and receive more hugs. Play with the above suggestions and keep track of how your choices affect you. Now is the time to tune into your needs and how you choose to nourish yourself, instead of depriving yourself.

# *SOME OF MY FAVORITE RECIPES*

I will be the first person to tell you I am no Julia Child or Martha Stewart in the kitchen. However I do enjoy all the benefits from homemade foods. So I put together a few recipes for you that are quick, healthy and truly satisfying. When I cook at home, I choose to keep the dishes on the mild side so my family and guests can season them with whatever tickles them at the moment. This way we are never bored with our meals and no one complains about the taste. So I encourage you to play with your food. Find you tasty bliss at each meal and have fun!

## Snacks, Juices & Smoothies *(OH MY!)*

### Butternut Squash Chips

1 small butternut squash (use long neck only)

olive oil

sea salt

Heat oven to 450 degrees. Cut squash into thin coin rounds. Spray or massage on olive oil and sprinkle with sea salt. Cook each side for about 10 minutes (longer if your rounds are not very thin). Let cool after each side is cooked and enjoy!

### Kale Chips

1 to 2 bunches kale Olive oil

Preheat oven to 425 degrees. Remove kale from stalk, leaving the greens in large pieces. Place a little olive oil in a bowl, rip your fingers and rub a very light coat of oil over the kale. Place kale on baking sheet and bake for 5 minutes or until it starts to turn a bit brown. Keep an eye on it as it can burn quickly. Turn the kale over and bake with the other side up. Remove and serve.

*Play with this recipe.* Use different kinds of kale or collard greens. For added flavor sprinkle with a little salt or spice, such as curry or cumin after rubbing on olive oil...or sprinkle with Brewer's Yeast for a slightly 'Cheesy" taste.

### Cucumber Raita

2 slicing cucumbers, peeled, seeded, and grated or chopped

1 cup plain nonfat yogurt

1 teaspoon chopped fresh mint leaves

1/4 teaspoon ground cumin

Press the cucumbers through a strainer to remove some of the water. Combine with the other ingredients and enjoy with pita chips!

### White Bean Puree`

| | |
|---|---|
| 1/2 t lemon juice | 1T sour cream |
| 3-4 T olive oil | 3/4 T cumin |
| 3/4 T chili powder | Salt to taste |

1 can organic white beans (cannelloni or white northern)

1 head roasted garlic-all garlic squeezed out (To roast garlic simply cut top of a head of garlic off and drizzle olive oil on it. Then wrap in tin foil and cook in oven at 400 degrees for 30 minutes)

Add all ingredients into blender and drizzle in olive oil until smooth. Chill in Fridge for 1 hour and serve with sprig of parsley and cumin sprinkled on top!

Easy Black Bean Dip

1 can Eden Organic Black Beans

1 Jar Organic Salsa

1/2 C Organic Corn

Combine all ingredients into bowl and garnish with cilantro then serve.

# Juice It Up...

Juicing is an incredibly effective way to cleanse the body, especially green juices! Green juices contain high levels of chlorophyll a powerful phytonutrient which attaches to toxins and heavy metals and helps remove them from your body. It also increases your blood's oxygen-carrying capacity by stimulating red blood cell production, and is fabulous for fighting off the negative effects of stress on the body.

Simply take any of the combinations I have listed below and put them into your juicer. They make a great snack, a wonderful short term program on their own (with supervision) and a wonderful afternoon pick-me-up instead of coffee or candy bars!

Some of my most favorite simple green juice recipes include:

• Celery, lemon, apple and ginger

• Celery, cucumber, lemon and apple (or pear)

• Celery, cucumber, kale, lemon and apple (or pear)

• Celery, cucumber, lemon, parsley, kale and green apple and pear

Remember keep the focus on getting as much greens as possible. Having a sweet fruit juices is ok, just not in excessive amounts.

## Smoothie Me!

<u>Sweet Avocado Smoothie</u>*(make in high powered blender or food processor)*

1/2 cup crushed ice

handful of kale

1/2 avocado

1 cup water

5-6 frozen pineapple cubes

honey to taste

Add in kale, ice, pineapple cubes, water and avocado. Blend on high speed setting for a few minutes until you no longer see parts of kale spinning around. This can be made thicker, and eaten with a spoon as a dessert, or thinner and served in a glass with a straw.

## My Morning Snack Smoothie

1/2 cup organic blueberries

1/2 cup organic strawberries

1/2 cup organic Blackberries

1/2 cup vanilla almond milk

Place all ingredients into blender then blend until done. Yummy!

*Meal Suggestion- heat up your left over brown rice and place about 2–3 tablespoons of the smoothie over the brown rice for a fruity morning porridge!

# Soups

Many of my soup recipes can be used as more than simply soup. They can be used as a sauce to put over pasta, brown rice, quinoa or any other whole grain. They can also be used as a sauce to top off a fish dish, chicken dish, stir fry's or even as a salad dressing. The only limitation is your imagination!

## Dina's Creamy Carrot Soup

1 Bunch Carrots

1 Small Onion

1 Golden or Sweet Potato

1T Earth Balance

1T Bragg's Amino Acid or Tamari

Water to cover veggies

Add all ingredients into pot and cover with enough water to cover veggies. Place lid on pot and let it come to a boil. Once at a boil, take lid off and let simmer until all veggies are soft. Add some Bragg's Amino.

Once soft, blend all veggies with hand blender and enjoy! You could even garnish it with a sprig of parsley!

*Meal Suggestion-This is a great base recipe for a sauce over a whole grain such as millet or quinoa, with some broccoli or other green veggies mixed in.

### Non-Dairy Creamy Broccoli Soup

1 1/2 C Organic Chicken Broth (optional-veggie broth instead)

2-3 C Water

1/2 Large Yellow Onion (diced)

1 Pkg. Organic Frozen Broccoli

3/4 Sheet Nori (sea weed sheet found in supermarkets where they sell sushi)

1 Large Yellow Potato (diced)

3 T Earth Balance

Sea Salt/Pepper to taste

Put all ingredients into pot,except butter and salt, and bring to a boil. Then put on simmer and lightly cover until all ingredients are soft. Blend with Hand Blender and then add in Earth Balance and Sea Salt. Blend again and serve!

## No Cook Creamy Tomato Soup

3 organic beefsteak tomatoes

1 avocado

1T olive oil

1/2 C Fresh basil

Sea salt & pepper to taste

Place all ingredients into high powered blender or food processor and blend. Serve in bowl and enjoy!

*Makes for a great base of a raw pizza as well as sauce for cooked pasta too!*

## Creamy Cucumber Soup

1 Avocado

1 Cucumber (seeds removed to prevent burping)

Pinch or two of Sea Salt

1/2 - 1 C Water

Fresh Cilantro or Watercress

Fresh Dill

In Cuisinart add all above ingredients except for the water. Blend everything together steadily and slowly add in water until soup is the consistency you desire. Eat and enjoy!

# Breakfast

### Dina's Cozy Autumn Breakfast

1 organic apple diced

1-2 tablespoons of water

2T cinnamon

1 pinch salt

1T honey

Brown rice *(optional- Uncle Ben's 90 sec brown rice)*

In sauce pan put water and diced apples, let come to simmer then add salt, cinnamon, and honey. Cover and let simmer for 3-4 minutes or until soft. Turn off heat. Add in rice and let sit on stove for 2 minutes.

### Breakfast Broccoli Slaw Stir Fry

1 Handful of Broccoli Slaw

1 Handful Shredded Zucchini

1/2 C Thinly Sliced Sweet Onion

1/2 -1C Brown Rice, Quinoa or Brown Jasmine Rice

Pinch Sea Salt or 1t Bragg's Amino Acid

1T Earth Balance buttery Spread

Dash of Old Bay or Nutmeg

In pan melt Earth Balance over medium high flame, and then add in onions, zucchini, and broccoli slaw. Pour in Braggs's Amino Acid and seasonings. Sauté in pan until colors or veggies get bright (about 4 minutes). Add in Grain of your choice and let cook together for 2 minutes or so. Serve and enjoy!

### Tasty Breakfast Burgers

2 C Oats

2 C Water

Minced Apple

½ C Raisins

½ t Sea salt

Honey (to taste)

1 T Cinnamon

Place all ingredients in a large sauce pan and heat on low flame to a simmer or until thick. Let cool on stovetop or in fridge, then form into patties and heat on skillet just as you would a regular burger. Best when made into small mini-burgers.

# Lunch

### Green Wrap

3-4 leaves Bibb lettuce

Fresh Watercress

Avocado, sliced

Tomato, sliced

2 of Lightlife's Organic Smokey tempeh Strips

Organically Grown Alfalfa Sprouts

Place Bibb lettuce flat on plate. Place all ingredients onto on closest end of lettuce. Roll away from you until all food is enclosed. Eat and enjoy!

## Sunshine Confetti

zucchini, yellow squash, carrots, red pepper yellow onion (shredded)

1C Fresh Cilantro

2 heaping handfuls of broccoli slaw or broccoli

1 T Earth Balance 1 T olive oil

1/2T paprika

sea salt / pepper to taste

Sesame seeds

*Optional- grilled or steamed sea food is fabulous with this dish!*

In heated sauté pan add Earth Balance and olive oil. When Earth Balance melts, add in shredded vegetables, broccoli slaw, paprika sea salt & pepper; After about 3-5 minutes add in cilantro and quickly sauté together. Sprinkle on sesame seeds and with serve over Rice Pilaf, brown rice or Quinoa...Delish!

## Oat Burger

2 cup oats

2 cups water

Fresh Rosemary

Fresh Thyme

½ cup Bragg's Amino or Tamari

Pepper

Diced Yellow, green and red pepper

Diced Onion

Place all ingredients in a large sauce pan and heat on low flame to a simmer or until thick. Let cool on stovetop or in fridge, then form into patties and heat on skillet just as you would a regular burger. Best when made into small mini-burgers.

# Dinner

### Mama's Vegetarian Chili

1 pkg. smart ground

sea salt/pepper

2T olive oil

1medium green pepper

1 medium red pepper

1  16 oz can diced tomatoes

1 small can tomato paste

2t chili powder

1t cumin

1 small jar salsa

2C Corn

1 small sweet onion

1can cannellini beans

1 can black beans

1can red kidney beans

In  a large pot add oil, onions & peppers. Sauté 2 minutes then add smart ground, chili powder, cumin salt & pepper. Next, add in salsa, tomatoes, tomato paste, corn, and all the beans. Cover and simmer on low for 35-45 minutes. Serve with corn bread or on top of polenta triangles.

## Seafood Corn Chowder

3 fillets of Tilapia or Orange Roughy, diced

1 can lump crab meat

½ lb medium shrimp, deveined, peeled,diced

2-3 butter potatoes          1

C whole, organic milk

2C water

2T butter

1 red pepper, diced

4C sweet corn

2t Old Bay seasoning

1 green pepper,diced

2 stalks celery

2T unbleached flour


In large pot heat butter, onions ,celery, peppers, potatoes. Sauté 2 minutes then add flour to create a rue. Add cooking wine and water. Let come to a boil uncovered. Add 2 cups corn & milk  Simmer for 15 minutes or until all veggies are soft and mushy. With hand blender blend together until smooth. Add remaining corn, fish, salt and pepper to taste and Old Bay. Simmer for 20-30 minutes covered. Serve with parsley as garnish.

## Sweets & Such

### Dina's Sweet Tahini Treat

1 can of Tahini

3 oz of toasted sesame seeds 3/4 cup raw honey

optional- add 1T of melted dark chocolate to drizzle over the top of each ball or add int mixture.

Add all ingredients into glass bowl and blend. It should be the consistency of play dough. Place in freezer for 30-40 minutes. Then roll into small balls.

Place in freezer again for 30 minutes then serve. To store keep refrigerated.

### Choco-Nut Crispies

1/2T organic butter

1 cup brown rice syrup

1/2 cup smoothe almond or cashew butter

1/2 cup dark chocolate chips

3 cups brown rice crispies cereal

Heat butter, brown rice syrup and nut butter in a large skillet, over low heat until creamy. Stir in the chips until they melt. Remove from the heat and stir in rice crispies. Gently press into a baking dish and allow mixture to set until firm, about 30 minutes. Cut into squares and enjoy.

# A FEW FINAL WORDS...

As you can see now, the real key to putting an end to mindless emotional stress eating and over eating lies in untangling ourselves from the exhaustive stress we live with every day and developing greater self awareness. Stress is a part of life, however we have the choice whether it takes over our lives, or if it's short lived. By being aware of our unique needs, slowing down and for a moment and showing ourselves patience, compassion and kindness, we begin to cut away at the anxiety filled "what if" "have to" "should" "must" and "have" thoughts that leads us down the spinning whirlpool of chaos we get so accustomed to living in. I believe in you and in your amazing ability to love yourself and make choices that uplift, empower, center and nourish you.I know that by applying many of the actions steps I've shared with you within the pages of this book, you now have a few tools at your disposal to untangle yourself from stresses clutches.

There is a big difference between selfishness and self-centeredness. Many of the women I work with have been taught that to take time and do something for themselves means they are being selfish. That if they spend time thinking about what they need first and take pride in themselves, they are being narcissistic. I believe by now you would agree that this would be a false understanding. If more women learned to make themselves a priority in a loving way through self awareness and positive inner self TALK, they would be able to give more fully to those they love and to their jobs as well as enjoy their lives more completely. What I have shared with you can help you do just that. One small step at a time. Again, stress is a fact of life. However it doesn't have to determine who we are or who we become. When we take back our inner power to live with self-awareness, self-worth and make mindful choices that truly nourish us at our very core, all that is toxic and burdensome simply falls away. I am living proof of this and so are the many women I've helped over the years.

If after reading this book you would like more support putting pieces of the puzzle together for yourself, I would be happy to help. I invite you to talk with me to find out if the same Hand-in-Hand coaching I talk about in the book is right for you. Please feel free to contact me to set up a consultation or check out one of my websites for more information.

DinaHansen.com

MindfulStressSolutions.com

Namaste`

Dina

# ABOUT THE AUTHOR

Dina Hansen is a Doctor of Natural Health who focuses on how our mind/body connection can help us get better control of stress, anxiety & mindless emotional eating habits. She lives in the Tampa Bay area of Florida with her husband, their daughter Raina and 3 funny cats named Lucy, Maggie & Katie Kat.

Through her own suffering, trials and education, she's discovered a more mindful path to creating authentic nourishment & balance for the whole person. A path that awakens the mind-body connection, allowing each individual to shine their light and satisfy their unique needs in accordance to their highest good. She guides women from all walks of life towards this balance through various forms of wholistic stress management coaching, live speaking events, self-paced programs, retreats and more.

You can learn more about her and her programs at:

DinaHansen.com
MindfulStressSolutions.com

52117305R00077

Made in the USA
Charleston, SC
11 February 2016